OCR→

D0638573

HEMP
FOR HEALTH

HEMP
FOR HEALTH

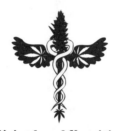

The Medicinal and Nutritional Uses
of Cannabis Sativa

Chris Conrad

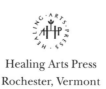

Healing Arts Press
Rochester, Vermont

Healing Arts Press
One Park Street
Rochester, Vermont 05767
www.gotoit.com

Note to the r eader: This book is intended as an informational guide. The remedies, approaches, and techniques described herein are meant to supplement, and not to be a substitute for, professional medical care or treatment. They should not be used to treat a serious ailment without prior consultation with a qualified healthcare professional.

Library of Congress Cataloging-in-Publication Data

Conrad, Chris
  Hemp for health : the medicinal and nutritional uses of Cannabis sativa / Chris Conrad.
    p. cm.
  Includes bibliographical references and index.
  ISBN 0-89281-539-6
  1. Cannabis—Therapeutic use. 2. Hemp. I. Title.
RM666.C266c66 1997
615'.32345—dc21   96-51628
                                                    CIP

Printed and bound in Canada

10 9 8 7 6 5 4 3 2

Text design and layout by Kristin Camp
This book was typeset in New Baskerville with Amvet as the display typeface

Healing Arts Press is a division of Inner Traditions International

Distributed to the book trade in Canada by Publishers Group West (PGW),
      Toronto, Ontario
Distributed to the health food trade in Canada by Alive Books,
      Toronto and Vancouver
Distributed to the book trade in the United Kingdom by Deep Books,
      London
Distributed to the book trade in Australia by Millennium Books,
      Newtown, N. S. W.
Distributed to the book trade in New Zealand by Tandem Press,
      Auckland
Distributed to the book trade in South Africa by Alternative Books, Ferndale

Contents

To the patients, practitioners, and nonviolent medical marijuana prisoners of the Drug War; to those who worked on or voted for Proposition 215; to the cannabis buyers clubs; to my wonderful wife, Mikki Norris; to my friends and family, and all who provided me with information and support to do this work; to my fellow researchers; to my mother, Betty Conrad; and to my father, Robert Conrad, who on his deathbed with cancer asked me to help others learn about and have access to medical marijuana when they need it.

Acknowledgments

Special thanks to Michael and Michelle Aldrich, Americans for Medical Rights, Maria Bruce, Business Alliance for Commerce in Hemp, Californians for Medical Rights, Cannabis Action Network, Bhagwan Dash, Rick Doblin, Drug Policy Foundation, Don and Jennifer Duncan, Family Council on Drug Awareness, Tom Flowers, Lester Grinspoon, Hash-Marijuana-Hemp Museum, Hemp Flax, Hemp Industries Association, Human Rights 95, Rowan Jacobsen, Keith, Ellen Komp, Steve Kubby, Ed Kunkel, Richard Lee, Marianne, Marijuana Policy Project, Raphael Mechoulam, Tod Mikuriya, Carol Miller, MontyPat, Multidisciplinary Association for Psychedelic Studies, Elvy Musikka, Ethan Nadelmann, Mikki Norris, Lynn and Judy Osburn, Candi Penn, Dennis Peron, Robert Randall, Brownie Mary Rathbun, Virginia Resner, Richard Rose, Eric Skidmore, Eric Sterling, Jeffrey Stonehill, Pet Sutton, Kirk Warren, Don Wirtshafter, Caroljo Woodnymph, Kevin Zeese, and George Zimmer.

A Note to the Reader

This book contains information concerning the healing properties of the plant *Cannabis sativa* L., also known as true hemp or marijuana. It is not a substitute for medical advice or treatment, and is only meant to inform the reader of available research regarding the many applications of this fascinating plant. Cannabis is used to treat symptoms, but is not a direct cure for most of the serious maladies described herein. It is a valuable adjunct for treatment and as part of a long-term health maintenance program.

No medicine is perfectly safe for every person in every situation. No medicine works equally well every time. Dosages and potential side effects vary according to body weight, metabolism, and a wide variety of other circumstances. Healing Arts Press urges extreme caution and careful monitoring of your reactions to any medicine you ingest. While self-medication with resinous cannabis is unlikely to have any serious negative consequences, always consult with a qualified health-care professional before using this or any other treatment for symptoms that may require full diagnosis and medical attention.

Although readily available, cannabis is illegal in most places throughout the world. The worst dangers of medical marijuana come from this illegal standing. Patients risk arrest, imprisonment, and loss of home, family, and dignity at the hands of law enforcement.

Introduction

What plant has been more studied, yet remains more mysterious, than the useful herb *Cannabis sativa?* There is a vast wealth of research, information, and conjecture available, along with a few overblown claims and outright falsehoods. An objective evaluation of cannabis was recently stated by the prestigious scientific journal, the *Lancet:* "The smoking of cannabis, even long term, is not harmful to health. . . . Sooner or later politicians will have to stop running scared and address the evidence: cannabis *per se* is not a hazard to society, but driving it further underground may well be."[1]

Large pharmaceutical companies have developed medicines with cannabis extracts, and even today some will admit that its use as medicine would doubtless be common if not for legal barriers. Eli Lilly makes a synthetic copy of a major active compound produced by cannabis, and even the Merck pharmaceutical company has recognized that "The chief opposition to the drug rests on a moral and political, and not a toxicological foundation."[2]

The *Journal of the American Medical Association* recently ran a commentary stating, "We are not asking readers for immediate agreement with our affirmation that marihuana is medically useful, but we hope they will do more to encourage open and legal exploration of its potential. The ostensible indifference of physicians should no longer be used as a justification for keeping this medicine in the shadows."[3] This book hopes to shine some light into some of those shadows by discussing the medical merit and therapeutic applications of cannabis hemp. This herb works as a natural medicine in a variety of ways that are all supported by both personal case histories and clinical scientific data.

People have used hemp in myriad forms. Its value is renowned. As measured by the amount of paper it has yielded over the millennia of commerce, or by the amount of paper used to tally its great contributions to history, it is hard to surpass the humble hemp plant. Hemp is a farm crop that has played a prominent role in 10,000 years of human industry and enterprise. Hemp has been familiar throughout history for its lush foliage crowded along riverbanks and its enormous production of fiber and oil in the fields of Eurasia, as one great civilization after another rose and fell. Each and every year, farmers and herbalists counted on the pattern of changing seasons to grow enough hemp for them to survive into the next era. Hemp was a part of the natural cycle of renewal and restoration.

Medical marijuana has demonstrably improved the lives of many people in varied and sometimes unlikely ways. Only for the past sixty years or so has there been a protracted campaign to suppress the facts about cannabis and deprive people of access to the hemp plant. Research has been stymied by government interference. Today, with thousands of new, legal medical users and millions of regular social consumers, people need a general reference manual to consult. *Hemp for Health* is intended to be such a book.

In the following pages, I discuss the direct applications of cannabis in the healing arts, as practiced in the allopathic, herbal, homeopathic, and ayurvedic disciplines. When all these applications are taken into account, it becomes abundantly clear that there is a place for hemp drugs in the modern medical formulary. *Hemp for Health* is intended to be a helpful handbook for patient and health-care provider; a user's guide, as it were, to safe and effective self-medication using one of our most ancient and respected herbs. I urge caution in the use of cannabis, as with any other medicine. Please remember that any effects produced, positive or negative, will only be temporary. If any significant problems occur, simply discontinue the use of cannabis and seek further medical advice. You and your personal physician are best equipped to determine which therapies work best.

THE ART AND SCIENCE OF RESINATION

Millions of Americans now use cannabis regularly. Still, there has never been a truly satisfactory English-language designation for cannabis drugs, which present a distinct class of substance. Nor has there been an adequate term to describe the resin's acute psychoactive effects. Unfortunately, much of the public discussion skips over this very basic and important concern, and relies on convenient points of reference to discuss cannabis, often with little regard for accuracy. For example, the term *intoxicant* biases our thoughts, and is otherwise misleading because cannabis is not toxic, having no practical lethal dose.

In the vacuum of a definitive term, cannabis consumers have coined their own words for its effects. In the vernacular of middle-class America, three words have gained widespread acceptance. Being *high* refers to a certain plateau of stimulated and pleasant mental awareness. Being *stoned* is the result of a stronger dosage in which the subject becomes more physically relaxed and mentally confused. Getting *wasted* means consuming more cannabis than is normally enjoyable or functional, which results in a sense of extreme tiredness and minor impairment. Unless you want to fall asleep, getting wasted is a waste of time.

A standardized terminology for cannabis drugs that eliminates language bias should be premised on an objective physiological characteristic. One common measure is the quality, quantity, and form of the resin taken from the female cannabis plant. The resin determines the intensity and nature of the psychoactive experience. Hence I use the term *resinous* effects, with *resin* as the root from which to grow new terminology.

The word *resinous* establishes a standard that describes both the organic substance and its psychoactive effect. The cannabinoids—the medical compounds in cannabis—occupy tiny trichomes on the resin glands that line the calyxes, hairs, and bottoms of the upper leaves and flowers of the female cannabis plant. A fortuitous similarity exists between the new term *resinate* and an existing English word, *resonate.* First, clinical research has identified an enhanced sensitivity to vibrations, such as tonal resonance, as being a dependable indicator of the onset of the effects of cannabis. Secondly, in a Hindu vision of the universe, an individual chants the resonant syllable *om* to attune to the harmonious vibrations of the cosmos. Since cannabis use is ingrained in Indian society, this analogy creates a link to a culture in which the use of cannabis is treated with respect, not fear.

Bear in mind that, whereas smoking cannabis on an occasional basis makes a person resinant, smoking cannabis on a constant basis to relieve chronic pain or another ongoing condition soon desensitizes the individual to the more pleasurable effects of the herb. Large allopathic doses establish a new base line for the patient, which soon becomes the norm. The federal IND allocation of ten cannabis cigarettes per patient per day is not a prescription for fun, it's a prescription for relief. Most medical users don't feel high, they just feel better.

A few people have expressed concern about the title of this book. "Shouldn't it be *Marijuana for Medicine?*" they ask. The truth is that *Hemp for Health* reflects the important bigger picture. Hemp is more than just marijuana, and there's much more to good health than merely taking medicines. Overall health is a result of many interrelated factors, such as nutrition, hygiene, exercise, environment, lifestyle choices, and necessary health care. The extraordinary hemp plant can contribute to almost all of these areas, in ways that may reduce the prevalence of many of the diseases now treated with marijuana. Hemp, in all its aspects, has been a key pillar of healthy societies for millennia. Thus, although much of this book focuses on the therapeutic benefits of marijuana, I wanted the title to take into account the greater role that *Cannabis sativa* can play in society.

I must stress that most types of *Cannabis sativa* do not have psychoactive properties. In writing this book, I use the term *industrial hemp* to refer to varieties of cannabis with no psychoactive effect. The terms *cannabis* and *hemp* refer to the entire genus, as they have for centuries. *Resinous cannabis* and *marijuana* refer to strains that produce a psychoactive effect. I hope that this standard will help the reader keep these distinctions clear.

Finally, I wish each of my readers a long and healthy life. Where appropriate, may hemp be a part of it.

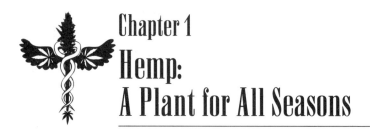

Chapter 1
Hemp:
A Plant for All Seasons

From a seed the size of a small pearl, a tiny shoot sprouts and a ten- to fifteen-foot plant grows in a few short months. Standing verdant green in its full splendor, hemp radiates its heady perfumes into the air. Left alone, the plant sheds its bloom and ripens its seeds, providing nutritious fare for the birds and beasts. Over the course of the winter, the cold, wind, and moisture tear at the outer bark and break free fibrous strands that hang off the inner wood when spring comes back around. At some transformational moment in history a flash of insight came to our human ancestors. Hemp's bark fiber was carefully gathered and twisted into cordage, combed into threads, and woven and sewn into garments. Hempseeds were gathered for food, then as the seed stock for next year's bounty. Although the life of a single hemp plant endures only a few months, its lineage has left a mark on human history throughout the ages.

Until recently, hemp was one of the most popular and highly valued crops in human society. Today it appears to be making a comeback. While its name has been borrowed by many lesser fiber crops, hemp remains a unique plant. It is a member of the botanical order *urticales*, which includes the hops plant *(Humulus lupulus L.)* used to make beer. It is usually placed in a distinct family called *cannabaceae*, although some prefer to assign it to *moraceae,* which includes the mulberry.[1] Botanists debate whether cannabis has several species or just one; however, since all varieties of cannabis crossbreed to produce fertile, hybrid offspring, they are generally all classified as one species with at least one major subspecies. It has scores of identifiable seed lines, or cultivars, and hundreds of regional names.

The plant's official scientific name is *Cannabis sativa* L., derived from the Greek *kannabis* and the Latin *sativa,* meaning "useful." This double name was first listed in A.D. 60 by Dioscorides and adopted by Carl Linnaeus for his 1753 compendium, *Species Plantarum.* A 1783 encyclopedia listed *Cannabis indica* as a separate species, named to honor India, the presumed homeland of this short, stocky, and highly resinous variety.[2] *Cannabis ruderalis* is a third variant, extremely hardy but with little commercial value.[3]

Hemp is a hardy herb that grows anew from seed each year.[4] The annual typically reaches heights of one to five meters (three to sixteen feet) in a season. It has a rigid central stalk that is rounded or slightly squared, more or less fluted lengthwise, with nodes at intervals where the leaves attach.[5] Its slender, woody stems range from six to twenty millimeters ($^1/_4$ to $^3/_4$ inch) in diameter, and its bark contains long bast fibers. When hemp grows in tightly crowded circumstances, as when farmed as a fiber crop, by season's end the mature plants have lost almost all their branches and foliage except near the very top. When given room to stretch its limbs, as when grown for seed or medicine, cannabis produces many strong branches along a central stalk that is three to six centimeters in diameter (one to two inches) with rough bark at the base. Side branches emerge just above the leaf nodes and spread out, giving the mature plant its distinctive, Christmas-tree shape.

The familiar, palmate hemp leaf is compound, with five to eleven leaflets. These leaflets are rich green on top and slightly lighter on the underside. Each fingerlike blade has serrated edges

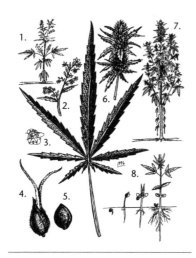

Cannabis sativa L.
1. Flowering male plant
2. Male flowers
3. Cannabis leaf
4. Female flower with stigmas extended
5. Fruit/hempseed
6. Female bud
7. Flowering female plant
8. Early growth

and is tapered at both ends. The central blade of each leaf grows to be five to fifteen centimeters long (two to six inches) by one to three centimeters wide ($^1/_4$ to one inch).[6] A wider blade is characteristic of *indica* seed lines; slender blades characterize *sativa*. *Indica* plants are also typified by shorter, densely branched stalks with thick, tropical foliage. Leaves grow in lateral opposite pairs arranged on alternating sides of the stem, except toward the ends of branches, where solitary leaves begin to switch sides preparatory to producing flowers. This change in pattern makes it possible to tell if a plant was grown from seed (which follows a regular leaf progression) or is a clone taken from upper stem cuttings (which have the irregular pattern). Most nutrients used by the growing plant are stored in its foliage and, if mulched, return to the soil at the close of the season.[7]

Each ovary develops a single seed in its own pod: a tiny, smooth, egg-shaped kernel, or *achene*.[8] These oil-rich fruits grow together in thick clusters along the flowering stalk. Immature seeds are pale green. Mature seeds range in color from dark gray to light brown and mottled, with dark seeds generally being much heavier than pale ones. When grown for seed, about half the dry weight of the female plant will be fruit. The seed portion is a variable, but the relative proportions by weight of the other parts, thoroughly air-dried, are fairly stable at approximately 60 percent stem, 30 percent foliage, and 10 percent root.[9]

INDUSTRIAL HEMP IS NOT MEDICAL MARIJUANA

Whereas only recently the idea was popularized that the resinous subspecies of hemp should be referred to as *Cannabis indica,* today we have the opposite emerging concept that the non-psychoactive varieties comprise a de facto subspecies commonly referred to as industrial hemp.

Each part of the hemp plant has special characteristics and distinct uses. Its stalk wraps one of nature's longest and strongest soft fibers around a woody core containing about one-third cellulose $(C_6H_{10}O_6)$—the organic compound used to manufacture paper, plastic, film, rayon, etc. The seed of the hemp plant is a complete and highly digestible source of nutrition for humans and animals and is also the source of a valuable oil. Its leaves and roots build, aerate, and otherwise improve the soil.[10] Industrial hemp requires no pesticides, and growing hemp can even clear fields of weeds without any herbicides. It can be fertilized using a combination of manure and rotation with nitrogen-fixing crops instead of chemical fertilizers. Due to its rugged nature, industrial hemp is an excellent crop for organic farming. With its myriad of commercial applications for its fiber and oil, industrial hemp offers exceptional economic value to farmer and manufacturer alike, with no potential for drug abuse.

Psychoactive drug content tends to be quite low in industrial seed lines grown in temperate climates. The cannabinoid compounds are most heavily concentrated in the female flower. A Dutch study of drug content in the flowers of two hundred hemp cultivars found ninety-seven varieties in the range of 0.06 to 1.77 percent tetrahydrocannabinol (THC), the psychoactive drug found in marijuana. Street-grade marijuana seized in the United States has hovered around 3 percent THC since 1982,[11] and medical grade should preferably be 4 percent or more.[12] The dense, industrial planting patterns lower the drug potency of even the most potent seed lines to minimal levels.[13] The competition for sunlight directs

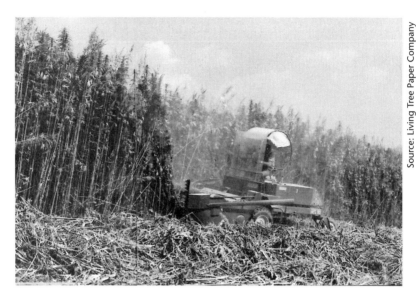

Industrial hemp crop in Spain.

Source: Living Tree Paper Company

energy away from producing resinous compounds and toward producing a taller, stalkier plant. Furthermore, industrial hemp is often harvested before the crop goes to flower and its resin flow becomes most potent. Seed selection for low-THC hermaphroditic cultivars allows for an easy visual distinction, since the male and female flowers are intermingled on the same stalk, rather than isolated on separate plants.

An early 1970s study proved that hemp grown for fiber is particularly low in THC.[14] Researcher Gilbert Fournier, commenting on the leaves and flowering tops of French monoecious (hermaphroditic) hemp, estimated that for "a minimal inebriant effect, one would have to smoke all at once 50 to 100 cigarettes of fiber hemp in order to obtain this effect."[15] Furthermore, there is essentially no THC in the stalk, seeds, or roots.[16] The nonpsychoactive compound cannabidiol (CBD) is relatively high in fiber hemp but low in marijuana, which makes industrial hemp doubly useless for smoking, because CBD actively blocks the psychoactive effects of THC.

Nevertheless, the leaves and flowering tops of certain cannabis plants do produce an attractive, aromatic herb. These seed lines are bred specifically for the therapeutic and spiritual value of their resinous female flowers. These "buds" produce an effective natural medicine comprising some sixty unique and therapeutically active organic compounds, along with a mild psychoactive substance. The human brain has special binding sites to which at least one cannabis compound, THC, attaches. These receptors are a unique part of our genetic design that put the human mind and the cannabis plant into direct contact.[17]

CANNABIS FLOWERS

Hemp sexuality is highly evolved. Cannabis is *dioecious*, meaning it has two completely separate flowers. About half the plants emerging from any batch of seeds will be male, and the remaining half female. Pollen-bearing, staminate male flowers occur in certain plants, while seed-producing, pistillate female flowers bloom on their own plants. Individual plants do occasionally become monoecious, especially during times of stress.[18] However, even specially bred monoecious seed lines tend to revert back to their dioecious ways over the course of a few seasons, and these hybrids have to be crossbred every year or two from the original dioecious genetic seed stock.

In the case of cannabis, the sexes are not created equal. The male is smaller, less vigorous, and has a shorter life span, serving primarily to pass on genetic material. Since the female blossom appears to the inexperienced eye to be little more than a thick leaf cluster atop the stem, it is the male plants that have often been called "flowering hemp." Their staminate flowers do look more like traditional blossoms with five greenish yellow or purplish sepals set in small radiating pod clusters hanging along the upper branches. At maturity, these pods burst open, and five stamens release a light and powdery pollen that is carried over a wide area on the wind. This thick, dusty pollen, a source of hay fever and allergies, adheres to the sticky resin excreted by the female flower. Once captured, it fertilizes the ovaries so the female plant can go to seed. Males die soon after their pollen is shed; the females remain green and vigorous for two months longer while the seeds develop.

Each individual female flower is a small, green, solitary, stemless blossom. It consists of a *calyx*—a thin, green, pointed pouch with a slit along one side; a pod that is nearly closed around the ovary except where two small white stigmas project through its apex to catch any passing pollen. The stigmas look like starched white threads poking up, and sometimes turn rusty orange as the flower ripens and matures. As the flowers grow, they become so tightly crowded together that they come to look like a thick, spiked club or a dense tangle of matted fur. This is why the flowering upper branches of cannabis are sometimes called by the Spanish word for an animal's tail, *cola*. Nestled together at the base of the small leaves near the ends of the branches, the flowers form tight clusters known as "buds." They are not, however, a traditional bud in the sense of a bloom that has not yet fully matured and opened into a flower.

If the flowers catch pollen and fertilize their ovaries, seed development becomes the major focus of plant activity. This diverts energy away from resin production and adds weight to the herb without increasing its drug content, so pollination is not desirable from a pharmaceutical standpoint. Cannabis grown for unseeded flower is called *sinsemilla*, Spanish for "without seed." Seedless cannabis is not a genetic fluke, like seedless grapes or seedless watermelon; it is simply unfertilized. Since there are no seeds produced, this is the most potent form of marijuana in proportion to its weight, and it generally has the highest market value as long as it is properly cured and manicured.

Tiny mushroom-shaped trichome glands, concentrated on the upper leaves and female flowers of cannabis, contain many of the medicinal compounds. On the more potent varieties of cannabis, these resin glands coat both the calyx and the pistil-

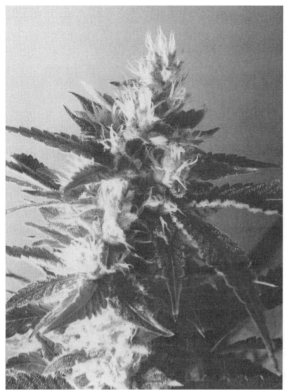

Photo: Rev. Hemp

Female cola

late hairs, glistening like sparkling, frosty crystals. Within them lie many of the healing chemicals discussed in this book: the resinous herbal compounds.

These compounds, in their natural raw form of medical marijuana, are a traditional and clinically proven form of therapy that is safe, effective, and affordable. We will look at what these chemicals are, how cannabis works, what concerns must be addressed regarding consumption and safety, and what all this means to the patient and to society in general. These are questions which have resonated through the ages, and which have gained new immediacy as the movement to legalize cannabis as medicine gathers momentum.

We stand at a threshold of understanding. The future is wide open.

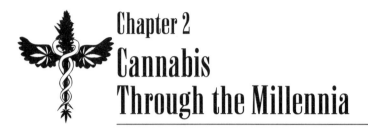

Chapter 2
Cannabis
Through the Millennia

As the Hindu poet Kalidasa wrote, "All things which are old are not necessarily true; all things which are new are not necessarily without fault. To the wise men, both of them should be acceptable only if they stand to the test."

Medical use of cannabis has stood the test of human history, and cannabis is mentioned in most ancient and medieval medicinal texts. Formulas containing hemp's seed or flowering tops were frequently recommended for difficult childbirth, menstrual cramps, rheumatism and convulsions, earaches, fevers, dysentery, epilepsy and insomnia, as well as to soothe nervous tension, stimulate appetite, and serve as an analgesic and aphrodisiac.[1] Although some of its applications are different today, in many respects we can learn much from the traditional use of cannabis hemp.

The oldest confirmed medical use of cannabis was in China. In 3750 B.C. China was a land ruled by petty warlords who sometimes protected and sometimes pillaged the peasants who labored on the land and filled the ranks of their armies. Beginning in the late Stone Age, villagers had begun to build walls to protect their communities from marauding bands of soldiers. At about that time, a series of heroic leaders arose and brought civilization to

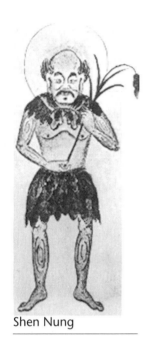

Shen Nung

the region. Among them was a philosopher farmer. His name was Shen Nung, and among his great contributions was teaching his people the value of the cannabis plant, *ta ma*. He taught the Chinese how to plant and harvest hemp, and how to use its seed in their diet. He taught them how to break fiber from the stalk and make yarn into fabric for clothing and sails; how to make traps to capture game; how to make nets for fishing and fowling. He led them into an era of commerce and prosperity.

Shen Nung became a mighty—indeed, mythic—emperor. Legend tells us he made it a point to record the healing arts. He collected traditions that had been handed down for generations so that medical knowledge could be shared from region to region and from one generation to the next. He produced the first reported pharmacopoeia, the *Pen Ts'ao,* the original of which was lost but later reconstructed during the Han dynasty (206 B.C.–A.D. 220). This work listed true hemp, *ta ma,* among the "superior" immortality elixirs. The female plant was said to possess *yin* energy (as opposed to the male plant's *yang*) and was recommended for "female weakness," rheumatism, beri-beri, malaria, constipation, gout, and absentmindedness, among other ailments. Lacking an original manuscript, the date 3727 B.C. is commonly ascribed to the *Pen Ts'ao.* Modern historians dispute this date, and many consider Shen Nung himself to be a composite figure encompassing numerous historical entities. In some manuscripts, Shen is shown wearing animal skins, but at least one shows him dressed in cannabis leaves, with a curious smile on his face as he picks his teeth with a stem. His reputation survives in the names of several geographic regions of China, such as Shen Dong province. It is still common to find hemp growing as an important crop in these areas.

Another ancient Chinese physician, Hoa-Gho, mixed the resin with wine as a painkiller adminstered to his patients.

The earliest surviving Chinese recipes tend to rely more on hempseed than on the marijuana flower. If any significant amount of the flower surrounding these seeds became mixed in with the recipe, there is a good chance that various can-

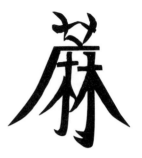

Calligraphy, *ma* (hemp)

nabis compounds were included in the resulting medicinal mixture. Nevertheless, the region does not have any strong history of using cannabis for its psychoactive properties. Its use was apparently limited to food, fiber, and medicine.

A GLOBAL MEDICINE

In the sixteenth century B.C., the Egyptian *Ebers Papyrus* recorded medical use of cannabis, which was also being used by the Coptics of Thebes in "smoke eating" incense rituals to communicate with God.[2] One of the earliest surgeons, Susruta, recognized in India in the third century b.c. that cannabis dried up mucous membranes, and he prescribed it as an antiphlegmatic. In addition to its varied religious and cultural uses in India, cannabis was used in Ayurvedic medicine for the alleviation of migraine headaches and stomach spasms, as an analgesic, antispasmodic, to promote digestion, and to assist in the flow of urine.[3]

In third-century B.C. Greece, Hippocrates, the "Father of Medicine," set aside the paranormal theory of health care and replaced it with a logical process. He recorded his case history observations along with the results of experimental procedures affecting the diet, emotion, occupation, climate, and environment of the patient. Through close observation, limited intervention, and systematic repetition, he was able to accurately di-

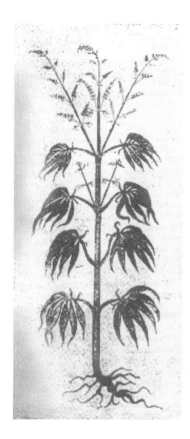

Roman drawing of cannabis from *Constantinopolitanus* (A.D. 500)

agnose and successfully treat the ill health of many clients. First he set about identifying a cause, and then devising a suitable cure. Hippocrates held that good health is a matter of balance between the outer world and the patient's inner being. This was achieved by combining special diets, exercise, bland drinks to stabilize body chemistry, wine to reduce stress, and botanical medicines, including purgatives and emetics, to flush the system. Building on this process, medicine made great strides during the classical era.

Dioscorides, the Roman Emperor Nero's private physician, praised the hemp plant for its commercial and medicinal properties and listed it as *Cannabis sativa*, the name it still bears.[4] Half a millennium later, the *Constantinopolitanus* gave us the oldest surviving botanical drawing of the plant.[5] In the second century, Pliny the Elder prescribed hempseed for constipated farm animals, the herb for earache, and hemp root poultices to ease cramped joints, gout, and burns.[6] His contemporary, Galen, added that hempseed "eliminates farting and dehydrates" and described how Romans would "fry and consume the seed together with other desserts."[7]

With the collapse of the Roman Empire and the suppression of knowledge during the Dark Ages, science was put on hold in Europe. The Inquisition brutally enforced its ban of the scientific method, herbal medicine, and anyone who strayed from the political orthodoxy of the medieval Church. Hygiene was a disaster. Health care once again degenerated into a mysterious domain of myth, magic, prayers, talismans, and spells to be cast or broken. Often, the prescribed treatment for any given disease was the drinking of some loathsome potion or the burning of a "witch."

Elsewhere, life went on in a more cultivated fashion. In China, herbal medicine and acupuncture became highly developed. Sophisticated medical procedures, including surgery, were being taught and practiced in India and parts of northern Africa. Information began to slowly filter back to Europe via the trade routes. Cannabis was discussed by Ibn Beitar in the thirteenth century at a time when Moslem sailors routinely used hashish to control their seasickness. This allowed them to travel by ship under weather conditions which might otherwise have kept them in port, and also helped them to achieve both their speedy conquest of the Mediterranean and their travel along spice routes to trade with India and distant areas of Asia. Hempseed is also discussed in great depth in the sixteenth-century Chinese manuscript *Pen T'sao Kang Mu* of Li Shih-chen. He compiled a variety of earlier writings and credited this seed with the power to increase the inner *chi* and slow human aging, stimulate and enhance circulation, increase the flow of milk in nursing mothers, and help those afflicted with paralysis. Li also said that using the seed to make shampoo would accelerate hair growth.[8]

During the European Renaissance, the veil of ignorance was slowly lifted after Leonardo da Vinci began to study the details of anatomy. The basis was laid for surgery. Diagnosis became more systematic and empirical. Diseases began to be enumerated, and treatments became more standardized. The development of the printing press to speed the flow of knowledge, the invention of faster ships to spur the European Age of Discovery, and the emergence of scientific methods to test the claims of folk tradition all came to prominence during this time period.

European explorers returning from Africa reported that Southern Rhodesians added cannabis to their herbal medicinal blends to treat malaria, blackwater fever, dysentery, blood poisoning, anthrax, and more, and that the Hottentots used hemp to treat snakebites and as a mood elevator.[9] Portuguese physician Garcia da Orta traveled to India to practice medicine, and there he became a student as well as a doctor. He selectively bred several strains of resinous cannabis, and in 1563 wrote a scientific treatise on its therapeutic uses.[10] The *Compleat Herbal*, a compendium published in 1645, recommends assorted cannabis preparations for hot or dry cough, jaundice and ague, fluxes, colic, worms and earwigs, inflammations, gout, "knotty joints," hip pains, and burns. [11]

The 1794 *Edinburgh New Dispensatory* notes that hempseed oil is added to milk to form an emulsion for treating coughs. It also reports therapeutic benefit in cases of "heat of urine" (venereal disease), and "incontinence of urine." The *Dispensatory* adds that, "Although the seeds only have hitherto been principally in use, yet other parts of the plant seem to be more active, and may be considered as deserving further attention." Twenty years later, Culpeper's classic pharmacopoeia, the *Complete Herbal*, summarized the medical uses of cannabis as known to him, including, "Being boiled in milke and taken, helps such as have a dry, hot cough," along with an extensive list of topical applications.[12]

When Napoleon invaded Egypt, French doctors went with his troops and soon began to investigate the medicinal value of cannabis. Its use was not limited to seeds and roots, or even to the raw foliage of the herb. This region, steeped in Moslem culture, was well aware of the psychological effects of cannabis, and artisans collected and pressed its sticky resin into potent, concentrated chunks of light blond or dark amber hashish. Growing, processing, and marketing the resin was a major commercial activity of the region, and the narrow alleys of Cairo were sweet with the fragrance of smoke wafting from the pipes of crafty merchants. Soldier and medic alike began to explore the dusty, twisting alleys and, nestled among them, the smoky hash parlors filled with cushions, couches, rich carpets, and tall hookahs. Soon they began to explore the resinous fumes that the locals seemed to enjoy so much as they drew deep breaths through long tubes attached to the water pipes.

THE AGE OF ENLIGHTENED CANNABIS USE

In the early nineteenth century, Western understanding of cannabis was on the verge of a great leap forward. As Europeans traveling in Africa and Asia came into contact with the resinous cannabis plants, scientific curiosity took its course. Physician Louis Aubert-Roche was among the first to investigate cannabis, with an 1840 book on using hashish to treat the plague, typhoid fever, and a variety of other physical ailments.

The curious subjective effects, such as time extension, inner dialogue, and a sense of awe, caused a stir in the newly emerging field of psychotherapy. Psychologist Jacques-Joseph Moreau de Tours took an interest in the mental effects of hashish in an era which finally viewed the human psyche in natural, humanist terms rather than as the uncontrollable supernatural domain of demons and angels. Through careful observation of people's reactions, including his own, to hashish—particularly their openness to suggestions and willingness to consider new possibilities—Moreau theorized that psychoactive substances could treat or replicate mental illness in a way to help cure patients. His 1845 studies on dhatura and hashish were prepared as a treatise that documented both physical and mental benefits, and ultimately led to modern psychopharmacology and the use of numerous psychotomimetic drug treatments.[13]

Around this same time, William B. O'Shaughnessy, the British East India Company surgeon in Calcutta, brought the telegraph to India and cannabis drugs to Britain. A keen observer as well as a ready and able scientific investigator, he introduced cannabis to Western medicine with an 1842 monograph on *gunjah.*[14] A graduate of Edinburgh Medical School in Scotland, he investigated this Hindu medicine systematically, experimenting with it on animals and patients, but also on himself, to ensure that he would have firsthand understanding of its effects. He validated folk uses of cannabis, discovered new applications, and ultimately recommended gunjah for a great variety of therapeutic purposes. O'Shaughnessy established his reputation by successfully relieving the pain of rheumatism and stilling the convulsions of an infant with this strange new drug. He eventually popularized its use back in England.[15] His most famous success came when he quelled the wrenching muscle spasms of tetanus and rabies with the resin. While he could not cure this man or other terminal patients, he did observe that the medicine reduced their symptoms of spasticity and their suffering, and allowed them to reappraise their circumstances and take on a dignified acceptance of their own mortality.

Since the temperate, industrial hemp crops of Europe did not have the same appearance or effects as the equatorial varieties, for some time scientists held that the resinous varieties called *Cannabis indica* were a distinct species from India. Few people understood the relation between the various cannabis cultivars. They understood that higher concentration of resinous drugs seemed to be connected to tropical growing conditions, but they did not know that the psychoactive, or psychotropic, effect is actually a result of several factors which at that time had gone largely unnoticed. The tetrahydrocannabinol (THC) in the resin acts as an ultraviolet light shield to protect the plants from the tropical sun. It also discourages many insect pests, so higher THC varieties survive better in times of pestilence. Also, centuries of seed selection had resulted in the development of more potent varieties of resinous cannabis, and other important differences occurred throughout the growing process. Male plants were removed, allowing female plants more room for branching, thereby producing a higher proportion of flowers. The plants were also heavily pruned, injured, deprived of water, and otherwise stressed by carefully trained growers to increase their potency. Since these practices were often tied to religious beliefs and practices, "objective" scientists from Europe had a difficult time giving them any credence, and Christian missionaries invariably rejected them as heresy.

Other climatic factors increasing resin production in cannabis were the result of the hotter temperatures and year-long equatorial light cycle, approximately twelve hours of daylight and twelve hours of dark—the perfect schedule for flowering the herb. In temperate zones, this pattern occurs only briefly and only twice per year, around the spring equinox and the fall equinox, so cannabis buds have less time to mature. Europe's colder weather and shorter flowering season significantly reduced the production of both flowers and resin. Greenhouses were still rare in Europe, and artificial grow lamps did not yet exist, so it was almost impossible to reproduce tropical conditions in temperate zones. Moreover, with a cheap and reliable source continuously available from the tropics, European scientists put little effort into producing resin from European hemp, which remained primarily a fiber and food crop.

Hashish had by then become a medication of international commercial interest, and scientific investigations moved to a global scale. Prominent physicians and pharmacists added cannabis to their medical arsenal to combat disease and human suffering. The *United States Dispensatory* first listed it in 1854, along with a cautionary note on the widely variable potency of the commercially available preparations. It noted that cannabis extracts "have been found to produce sleep, to allay spasm, to compose nervous inquietude and to relieve pain. . . . Complaints to which it has been specially recommended are neuralgia, gout, tetanus, hydrophobia, epidemic cholera, convulsions, chorea [spasticity], hysteria, mental depression, insanity and uterine hemorrhage."[16] The name Smith Brothers is still widely known for its cough medications. The Edinburgh-based family obtained a potent extract of *indica* in 1857 that became the basis for innumerable tinctures well into this century. Further south, the highly respected Sir John Russell Reynolds served a thirty-year tenure as Queen Victoria's personal physician. During his extensive service, Reynolds found cannabis useful for treating menstrual cramps, dysmenorrhea, migraine, neuralgia, epileptic convulsions, and senile insomnia. He wrote a scientific review of cannabis in 1890 that noted, "When pure and administered carefully, it is one of the most valuable medicines we possess."[17]

Other conditions for which cannabis drugs were often prescribed in the late nineteenth century were loss of appetite, inability to sleep, migraine headache, pain, involuntary twitching, excessive coughing, and treatment of withdrawal symptoms from morphine and alcohol addiction. At least one hundred major articles were published in scientific journals between 1840 and 1900 recommending cannabis as a therapeutic agent for various health conditions. Cannabis was also still widely used by herbalists and was a natural choice for the homeopathic tinctures that were popular. Reports in the literature described its effectiveness over a wide range of ailments, including gynecological disorders such as excessive menstrual cramps and bleeding, treatment and prophylaxis of migraine headaches, alleviation of withdrawal symptoms of opium and chloral hydrate addiction, tetanus, insomnia, delirium tremens, muscle spasms, strychnine poisoning, asthma, cholera, dysentery, labor pain, psychosis, spasmodic cough, excess anxiety, gastrointestinal cramps, depression, nervous tremors, bladder irritation, and psychosomatic illness.

By 1896 several useful new resin derivatives were developed. In a cooperative venture, Eli Lilly and Parke Davis developed a very potent domesticated *indica* strain called *Cannabis Americana.* Cannabis was also included in various mixtures, such as Brown Sequard's *Antineuralgic Pills.* At least thirty different pharmaceutical preparations contained cannabis, including Eli Lilly's *Dr. Brown Sedative Tablets, Syrup Tolu Compound,* and *Syrup Lobelia;* Parke Davis's *Casadein, Veterinary Colic Mixture,* and *Utroval;* and Squibb Co.'s *Corn Collodium* and *Chlorodyne.*[18] In the early twentieth century, hemp compounds were still common in corn plasters, veterinary medicine, and non-intoxicating medicaments. One researcher of the era noted, "extracts of cannabis were about the only compounds that could be used for pain relief and anxiety."

However, important changes had already occurred in the world of the medical practitioner: the development of morphine and the hypodermic syringe. The injection needle was now seen as the modern means to deliver medicine. Since cannabinoids are fat soluble, they cannot be dissolved in water or easily injected into the bloodstream for therapeutic benefit. This makes cannabis impractical—in fact, downright dangerous—to take by intravenous injection.[19] Hence the therapeutic use of cannabis began to decline and to be replaced with water-soluble, injectible pharmaceuticals. Cannabis preparations gradually disappeared from the turn-of-the-century apothecary for several reasons: Lack of injectible preparations, difficulty in obtaining standard potency batches, and the wide variability of individual responses to the same dose. Also important was the introduction of a multitude of synthetic drugs that were easier to produce in standardized forms, and more convenient for the physician to administer—although seldom as effective as, and usually much more toxic than, cannabis. Nevertheless, twenty-eight pharmaceutical preparations containing cannabis were still in use when virtually every use of the plant, including medical, was abruptly outlawed in the United States.

THE MARIHUANA TAX ACT OF 1937

The legislation that ultimately banned virtually all use of the hemp plant had its origins in the corrupt world of the post-prohibition federal Treasury Department. It came in the form of a special interest subsidy, disguised as a tax law. The Marihuana Tax Act of 1937 was designed to give a boost to the logging and synthetic fibers industries by eliminating industrial hemp from the market. The Du Pont company stood to make the most money off this legislation. Its archives report that the government had embarked on an experiment by which "The revenue-raising power of government may be converted into an instrument for forcing acceptance of sudden new ideas of industrial and social reorganization."[20] Two years later, without mentioning the ban on hemp, the corporate president bragged that "Synthetic plastics [made from mineral, chemical, petroleum, and fossil fuel deposits] find application in fabricating a wide variety of articles, many of which in the past were made from natural products."[21]

The trick was to rewrite the law by picking one of the plant's hundreds of street names and using that word as a smoke screen to hide the real effect of the bill. Americans were quite familiar with this plant under the names of *hemp* for industrial use and *cannabis* for medical use. But a flurry of newspaper stories with lurid headlines exagerated the problems of Mexican border towns, where locals were said to smoke an exotic and dangerous new drug known as *marihuana*. The Federal Bureau of Narcotics, faced with post-Prohibition budget cuts, seized the opportunity to boost its own importance by playing upon racist tendencies and stigmatizing both the plant and its users. They quietly redefined the obscure slang term to include all *Cannabis sativa* products, and carried a bill to Congress.

The tactic worked, even though it met some resistance. A major industrialist denounced the bill, pointing out that "The point I make is this—that this bill is too all-inclusive. This bill is a world encircling measure . . . the crushing of this great industry under the supervision of a bureau—which may mean its suppression."[22] The American Medical Association sent its top lobbyist to Congress to oppose the legislation. Dr. William C. Woodward charged that "We cannot understand yet, Mr. Chairman, why this bill should have been prepared in secret for two years without any initiative, even to the profession, that it was being prepared. . . . No medical man would identify this bill with a medicine until he read it through, because *marihuana* is not a drug . . . simply a name given cannabis." When the measure's passage was imminent, Dr. Woodward wrote a prophetic warning to the committee. "The obvious purpose and effect of this bill is to impose so many restrictions on the medicinal use as to prevent such use altogether. . . . It may serve to deprive the public of the benefits of a drug that on further research may prove to be of substantial value."

Woodward's words came true with a vengeance. The entrenched prohibition enforcement bureaucracy now had new prey to pursue. Doctors who prescribed cannabis or even dared study its effects were treated as criminals. Patients, physicians, farmers, and marijuana users were locked away with rapists and murderers. Once prohibition became the law of the land, the research of centuries past was cast aside. The popular press trumpeted one hysterical claim after another of "dangers of marihuana," yet the few scientific studies that were able to be done on cannabis found little harm and great potential for benefit. New York's 1942 LaGuardia Commission used the most sophisticated equipment and methodology available to examine and refute virtually every alleged health risk and psychological effect that had been reported to Congress to support marijuana prohibition. The drug police responded by destroying the careers of several reputable doctors who challenged them.

The fledgling Drug War was temporarily interrupted by the Second World War. The federal government organized patriotic farmers to grow a million acres of industrial hemp for the war effort, especially to supply the Navy and Air Force with rope, parachutes, and other essentials. Soon after the war, however, federal and state police cracked down again, this time targeting ethnic minorities and entertainers.

Throughout most of the twentieth century, medical marijuana had been largely overshadowed by the intense propaganda war raging around the plant's social use. Patients who claimed their conditions benefited from cannabis were routinely ridiculed and locked away. Research into cannabis and its medical uses continued to advance in a few countries, but international pressure tightened against it with the adoption of the United Nations Single Convention Treaty.

During the 1960s, marijuana use among youthful protesters politicized the issue. In a case involving Timothy Leary, the U.S. Supreme Court ruled that the Marihuana Tax Act was unconstitutional. In response, drug scheduling laws were written under President Richard Nixon, which were then used as a political weapon in the early 1970s. Industrial hemp was all but forgotten. Marijuana was officially declared to have no medicinal value. It was defined as a hallucinogen as a matter of bureaucratic convenience, and relegated to the category of prohibited drugs, Schedule 1. Nonetheless, when Nixon's conservative advisory committee studied the data and proposed ending criminal penalties on cannabis in 1972, it also described some possible medical benefits of the plant. A few patients successfully argued medical necessity defense cases in court, and the federal Investigational New Drugs program went into effect. This particular approach had the unfortunate side effect of nullifying official recognition of existing cannabis research, because it was now considered a "new" drug that had to start over from scratch. The law was a cruel hoax that pretended to allow medical access to marijuana, without requiring any controlled studies to be undertaken. No substantial numbers of patients were permitted to participate in the program, and the few who were enrolled had to first undergo criminal prosecution and prove their medical necessity. This lack of proper implementation was cited in 1991 as the main reason for ending the program.

CONTINUING RESEARCH AND DEVELOPMENTS

New interest in the medicinal history of cannabis began to rise in the 1970s. In 1973 Tod Mikuriya, M.D., a staff researcher for the Nixon commission, compiled some of the major medical works on cannabis into one book, *Marijuana: Medical Papers,*

1839–1972. Important new discoveries were still being made. In 1965, Dr. Rafael Mechoulam of Hebrew University in Jerusalem, Israel, isolated pure delta-1-trans-tetrahydrocannabinol (THC) and identified it as the principal psychoactive ingredient. This represented a new class of compounds, structurally different from other drugs, with demonstrable medicinal powers. After reviewing the latest data on cannabis, the U.S. Department of Health, Education and Welfare released a report in 1971 that acknowledged that "In the future, Cannabis or its synthetic analogs may prove to be valuable therapeutic agents."[23] During the 1970s at Pfiser Laboratories, researchers working with analogs of THC claimed to have produced synthetic analgesics one hundred times more potent than cannabis. Unfortunately, they also had a much stronger "high." The company eventually dropped its research because of this side effect, plus the economic reality that opiates, the true narcotics, already controlled the heavy-sedation market. Unlike a classical narcotic, cannabis does not knock a patient out; it only causes drowsiness and promotes sleep. Likewise, cannabis does not kill pain like an anesthetic; it reduces pain like an analgesic. Drug companies prefer a strong medication to a gentle remedy, and their economic interest in cannabis eventually diminished.

The scientific community eagerly explored the possibilities, and the National Institute of Drug Abuse (NIDA) held an important summit in November of 1975. Many of America's leading cannabis researchers attended the Asilomar Conference. Seminars and compiled reports indicated that cannabis and its extracts and analogs would probably return as one of the world's major medicines within a decade. The next year, Dr. Sidney Cohen and Richard Stillman published a hopeful prognosis for protocols and therapies using cannabis in numerous medical applications, entitled *The Therapeutic Potential of Marijuana.*

Unfortunately, hard-liners were back in firm control of research. Within a few years, permits and grants regarding marijuana were systematically perverted and politicized, and a clear pattern of bias has long since become familiar. By the late 1970s propaganda had once again replaced science in the mechanisms of government claims, and the scheduling issue that would allow doctors to prescribe medical marijuana was tied up in the courts.

Amid all the political maneuvering, some serious research has continued to be done, which has laid the groundwork for marijuana to gain informal acceptance within the medical profession. Continuing research verified the herb's value in treating migraine headache.[24] Dosage and consumption patterns were studied and evaluated, which demonstrated its relative safety for human consumption.[25] Studies were done on the effects that cannabis has on the eyes that verified its benefit in reducing intra-ocular pressure and thereby relieving the buildup of ocular fluids that characterize glaucoma.[26] Hollister demonstrated the value of cannabis as an appetite stimulant in 1971, and it has since been applied in the treatment of wasting syndrome associated with AIDS, anorexia, and cancer.[27] In 1980 Sallan documented its utility in controlling nausea and vomiting, which led to its use in offsetting the debilitating effects of chemotherapy undergone for cancer or AIDS.[28] Clinical studies combined with abundant anecdotal evidence and the direct observation of physicians led a substantial part of the medical community to re-evaluate the therapeutic use of cannabis. In 1988 Vinciguerra corroborated the medical value of smoking marijuana.[29] In 1991 a Harvard University team found that 44 percent of the cancer specialists who responded to a survey had privately recommended to some of their patients that they smoke cannabis to relieve chemotherapy side effects. Forty-eight percent also said they would like to prescribe it in some cases, if it was legal, while 54 percent agreed that cannabis should be legal for doctors to prescribe.[30]

Research into the nonpsychoactive constituents of cannabis resin also made significant advances. Researchers used cannabidiol, or CBD, to produce antibiotics, and identified dose levels that measurably and significantly improved patient control in movement disorders, and reduced symptoms of epilepsy, multiple sclerosis, and Huntington's Disease.[31] The chemical relationships and interactions between the psychoactive and nonpsychoactive compounds in cannabis resin were even studied, with the surprising discovery that CBD enhances medical benefits but blocks the psychoactive effects of THC.[32] This characteristic was later applied in working with psychological illness.[33]

Meanwhile THC has been produced in a synthetic form by Eli Lilly and marketed under the generic name Dronabinol and the trade name Marinol. It has been prescribed for many of the same conditions that cannabis is used to treat, with varying results. A variety of other delivery systems have also been developed. An inordinate amount of attention has been directed at detecting inert cannabinoids in the hair, urine, and feces of users.

Recently, research has been directed at identifying the location and function of the physical mechanisms that bring about the cannabis resin's neurological effects.[34] It began with the identification of special receptor sites for cannabinoids within the human brain. Their locations were dutifully enumerated and charted. A subsequent study identified a simple protein binder, dubbed anandamide, that attaches the compound to the surface tissue of the brain. The implications of these discoveries are yet to be fully felt. We are just now coming to terms with how this information might be applied for the benefit of those who suffer from disease and chronic conditions, as will be discussed in the coming pages.

And so, humanity and cannabis once again stand together at a dawn of new potential. Where will the new day lead us? Chances are that we will get a pretty good idea by studying where we have traveled in the past. Cannabis is hardly a cure-all, but it is a terrific medicine and a valuable tool for the healing arts and sciences.

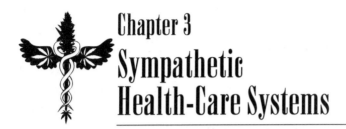

Chapter 3
Sympathetic
Health-Care Systems

Because there are a number of health-care systems that can accomodate cannabis use, it makes sense to take stock of the options before finalizing a therapeutic regimen. Conventional medicine as it is practiced today is known as allopathy. This term describes licensed, "orthodox" medicine, as practiced by a graduate of a medical school granting an M.D. degree. In this approach to treatment, health is considered to be the absence of disease. Hence, disease is an invader to be combated by taking a medication from the physician's arsenal and using it to annihilate the problem.

Important landmarks in the history of allopathy include 1666, when British physician Thomas Sydenham popularized the use of the cinchona plant, containing quinine, to cure malaria. In 1796 Edward Jenner observed similarities between the relatively benign disease cowpox and the deadly smallpox. This observation advanced health care to the realm of inoculations and laid the groundwork for modern immunology. Scientific advances branched out exponentially during the following two centuries. Robert Koch developed bacteriological techniques that proved the importance of controlling micro-organisms in the water supply. A keener understanding of the importance of sterile medical conditions, in surgery and elsewhere, quickened the pace of change. In 1805 morphine was developed, followed by cannabis drugs in 1842 and aspirin in 1899. Louis Pasteur produced a germ theory that included the use, in 1880, of true vaccines, and "pasteurizing" milk to kill bacteria and retard spoilage. In 1928 Alexander Fleming recognized the antibacterial power of penicillin, which clinched allopathy as the dominant medical paradigm.

Steadily improving technology and controlled studies came into play, but the prohibition of cannabis hurt the quantity and quality of research, and the attitudes of the medical and social communities as well. Unfortunately, the conventional orthodoxy has become more and more response driven and chemical oriented. The result is a massive dispensing of pharmaceutical pills, tablets, capsules, suppositories, and liquid medicines to be taken orally or injected intravenously. This practice is important and has enormously improved the health and well-being of millions of human beings, but at a terrible price. In recent decades, medical practice has fallen into the self-serving hands of multibillion dollar companies that profit from manufacturing and licensing these drugs, and of government agencies who both make up and administer the rules and regulations through which that profit is derived. The licensing process, originally designed to protect the public, has become so inept and corrupt that it stalls the release of certain drugs, especially natural remedies, while making available more costly and dangerous surgical procedures and pharmaceutical drugs. The physician is therefore left in the severely limited role of offering only the approved, expensive drugs and procedures. The patient passively consumes these in whatever amount and form the doctor indicates, and pays whatever price drug companies dictate.

HERBAL MEDICINE

Today's herbalists are leading a return to natural healing. They use the leaves, flowers, stems, berries, and roots of plants to prevent, relieve, and treat illness. Herbs tend to stimulate the immune system, rather than attack invading organisms. For example, echinacea, a common treatment for infection, does not work by killing germs directly, but by stimulating white corpuscle production within the blood stream. The body's natural defense system takes over from there. As a result, adverse reactions to herbs, if any, tend to be mild and can usually be eliminated simply by discontinuing use of the herbal medication and waiting for it to pass from the patient's system.[1]

From an orthodox standpoint, this approach is considered experimental but, in fact, it is probably our most traditional field of medicine. Witch doctors and shamans used herbs extensively in their practice. Primitive societies, including the few who have survived into modern times, maintain a close understanding of the subtleties and healing powers of the plant kingdom. Herbology was profoundly important in ancient China, including various uses of cannabis. Hieroglyphic instructions for herbal techniques were carved into temple stone in ancient Egypt, and cannabis incense smoke was "eaten" in the temples of Thebes to dispel demons.[2] Ashurbanipal prepared a record on clay tablets in 650 B.C. Babylon that chronicled the use of cannabis resin going back to even earlier times.[3] During the Middle Ages, the family herb garden was a backyard pharmacy, with instructions handed down by oral tradition from one generation to the next. When the British physician Nicholas Culpeper chose to step away from academics and become a community doctor, he prepared two books: *A Physical Directory,* in 1649, followed shortly thereafter by *The English Physician.* He organized his information for use by the lay person as well as the doctor. Much of the approach to medicine and the healing arts was then based on the idea that patients had to take some of the responsibility for being their own physicians.

The first *U.S. Pharmacopoeia,* published in 1820, relied heavily on herbology. Soon thereafter, the "snake oil" medicine shows led to such flagrant quackery that people became sick or even died after swallowing the potions. Often there was little more than ethyl alcohol in the medicine bottle. Although authentic traditional medicines remained quite effective, the federal government jumped in to regulate the industry, with unintended consequences. Large commercial drug companies soon gained a foothold and took control of both the private markets and the regulating bureaucracies. Drugs came to be patented and marketed by trade name. By the time the *U.S. Pharmacopoeia* was designated the official legal standard in 1906, many valuable remedies which had been common knowledge among our forebears were already being labeled unscientific, discarded as folklore, and banned from the doctor's bag.

Herbology, the historic mainstream of general medical practice, has since become marginalized and the healing arts privatized. Profits replaced patients as the dominant interest of the industry. Pharmacists have meticulously dissected and analyzed our medicinal plants. Certain "active" compounds have been isolated, extracted or synthesized, and authorized for a very narrowly focused chemical reaction. Botanical research has hit a point where many of our most effective prescription drugs are either derived from herbs or are chemical analogs— synthetic compounds modeled after organic compounds. Morphine, codeine, and a treatment for diarrhea, called paregoric, all come from the opium poppy. Atropine is a belladonna extract. Pseudo-ephedrine is a pharmaceutical version of ephedrine, a decongestant derived from the plant ephedra. Dronabinol is a synthetic copy of the THC found in natural cannabis. The traditional *Pharmacopoeia* has now been set aside and replaced with the *Physician's Desk Reference*. This contains an extensive inventory of approved chemically manufactured drugs, listing particular chemical compounds, recommended and lethal dosages, and specific actions of each drug—along with an extensive list of warnings, contraindications, and possible side effects. Individual molecules have been identified and patented. Still, not everyone is convinced that the single compound approach is the best system for medicine.

Modern herbalists recognize that the healing power of a plant lies in the interactions of all its various components. That includes the drug compounds, but also assorted minerals, vitamins, volatile oils, essential oils, glycosides, alkaloids, bioflavonoids, and other substances, both known and unknown. In addition to the registered "active" ingredients, herbs include buffers, detoxifiers, and synergistic compounds that can greatly enhance the safety and medical efficacy of the active compounds. It is this very complexity, which makes herbs so powerful, that also makes them difficult to standardize and regulate. This characteristic is then used as an excuse to suppress the use of medical herbs, with the marijuana laws being the most glaring example.

The value of medicinal herbs remains undeniable. Their therapeutic use is administered in numerous forms. These include raw natural herb, bolus, capsules, extract, lozenges, ointments, poultice, suppositories, syrups, tablets, teas or infusions, and tinctures. In the case of cannabis, the herb can also be smoked or prepared in food. Raw cannabis is often difficult to take in solid form, and should first be soaked in oil to release the cannabinoids. Tinctures are alcohol-based, concentrated extracts of active compounds taken from the herb, and sometimes have a very strong and unpleasant taste. Alcohol also acts to preserve the compounds and helps the body to assimilate them. If patients wish to reduce their alcohol intake, they can mix the appropriate dose with a few ounces of very hot water and wait a few minutes for the alcohol to evaporate before consuming the remedy. Extracts are similar to tinctures, but in a more concentrated form. They are sometimes made using water rather than alcohol to leach out the medicinal compounds and hold them in suspension. If the technical process concerns you, check the label on commercial products for details.

Unless they are concentrated, raw herbs tend to be significantly less potent than tinctures or extracts. Cannabis, in particular, should be heated to potentiate the effect of its synergistic compounds and help the body to assimilate them. This is another good reason to smoke, vaporize, or bake with it. Dried herbs can be ground up into powder and consumed in a gelatin capsule or a compressed tablet. They can be steeped in scalding hot water. The resulting infusion is sipped to allow the patient to savor the flavor, ingest the beneficial compounds, and increase overall fluid intake. This helps flush the system of toxins. Herbal extracts and essential oils can also be suspended in an inert base, such as corn syrup. This thick liquid can be taken in measured doses as a syrup, or solidified into a lozenge that is dissolved in the mouth and released over a period of time. Ointments, poultices, rubs, and salves are external applications that combine herbs and their extracts with a variety of oils, creams and other topical preparations. They are used to protect and heal broken skin, to fight infections, to soothe rashes, skin irritations, and aching muscles, and to reduce inflammations. Soaking in a hot herbal bath is a soothing, relaxing, and therapeutic experience.

HOMEOPATHIC REMEDIES

A whirlwind of controversy swirls around the use of homeopathic treatments. Nonetheless, many people have found relief in its practice, so it deserves mention here. Homeopathy was developed by the German physician Samuel Hahnemann (1755–1843) of Leipzig. It focuses on treating the specific symptoms of a medical condition rather than directly attacking the causes. Because symptoms can vary, the same disease may require a completely different treatment for one patient than it does for another, based on their individual symptoms and responses to various homeopathic preparations. This requires the physician to evaluate and attend to the specific needs of each patient in their unique situation. A homeopath may recommend changes of diet and lifestyle as part of the treatment. They prescribe certain drugs and make adjustments as they monitor the patient's progress. Following a homeopathic regimen requires patience to solve the problem, and sometimes six months or longer of treatment. While more time-consuming than some therapies, homeopathic remedies may offer an amazingly effective and gentle alternative to allopathic procedures.

Dr. Hahnemann made his initial discovery while in a healthy state. He determined to learn how the cinchona bark worked to relieve malaria—not merely to deduce the active organic compound, quinine, but to uncover the process behind the cure. He consumed some of the bark, and promptly developed symptoms of acute malaria. The doctor summed up his discovery as the law of similars: "like cures like." Through further experimentation, he came to the paradoxical conclusion that ingesting a minute, homeopathic dose of certain medicinal extracts can actually cause the reverse effect of taking a strong allopathic dose. He deduced that such remedies must stimulate the body's inherent "vital force" and increase the patient's ability to resist disease, somewhat like an inoculation.[4] This approach to healing reached its greatest popularity in the United States in the late nineteenth century, when 15 percent of the doctors here were homeopaths, and cannabis tinctures were common medicines.

Today homeopaths understand this process as a complex interrelationship of biological factors, such as the immune and regenerative systems, functioning within the setting of the patient's mind and body. As with any health-care system, the patient's confidence in both the doctor and the therapeutic regimen will ultimately affect the outcome of the treatment. Homeopathy respects the individuality of each patient and requires close observation of both the subject's obvious and subtle reactions. Homeopathic researchers often use self-administered doses of their remedies to experience and keep track of their own subjective and physiological reactions to the compounds before prescribing them to others.

Homeopaths report that the effectiveness of their medicines actually increases with successive dilutions of the medicinal substance. As long as the medicine is violently shaken between each dilution, the remedy becomes more potent. This unusual approach to potency is a controversial aspect of homeopathy. There is no scientific explanation for it, yet the effect has been documented around the world. The reliance on trace doses has led many conventional allopathic doctors to regard homeopathy as little more than a placebo effect presenting itself as a cure. However, it does bring relief to some.[5] Patient responses have been predictable enough for remedies to be prepared according to standards set by the *U.S. Homeopathic Pharmacopoeia.* Furthermore, a number of controlled studies have shown the efficacy of homeopathic medicine in treating various diseases.[6] A major review of the existing research on homeopathy, prepared by medical school professors at the request of the Dutch government, was published in the *British Medical Journal.*

CANNABIS IN HOMEOPATHY

A classical homeopath would not simultaneously prescribe to the same patient one medicine for a headache, a separate one for nausea, a third to help induce sleep, a fourth for depression, and so on. Instead, they identify a single medicine that covers as many symptoms as possible. Cannabis is an excellent source of homeopathic remedies, and it came into play as such early on. The following 1842 discussion on plant selection for preparing homeopathic tinctures of hemp drugs was based on an earlier German work. "We take the flowering tops of male and female plants and express the juice, and make the tincture with equal parts of alcohol; others advise only to use the flowering tops of the female plants, because these best exhale, during their flowering, a strong and intoxicating odor."[7] In light of modern research, we can see the importance of factors like the ratio of CBD-bearing male flowers to THC-bearing female flowers in predicting different effects and adjusting extracts to suit the situation. There are further significant differences in the acute effects of the two major cannabis types, which are reflected homeopathically. Variations in the cultivar's organic chemistry may explain the past difficulty of getting consistent reactions to cannabis extracts.

To determine which symptoms are likely to be affected positively by cannabis homeopathy, we need to know its chronic effects at massive doses. One of the most consistent and marked symptoms of cannabis use is the sensation of prolonged time. In addition, a peculiar separation of the mental faculties occurs, during which one functions as both a participant and an observer. Massive doses of resin can stimulate creative vision, so a homeopathic dose might be used to treat a patient with delusions or hallucinations, or to comfort someone having a difficult experience on LSD. Other problems which benefit from cannabis homeopathy are urinary infections, muscle cramps, backache, dry mouth, dry vagina, tremors, pneumonia, palpitations of the heart, and tinnitus, a pathological ringing in the ears. In general, extract of *sativa* is better for treating milder physical or mental problems. *Indica* is more effective for serious physical maladies. However, some mixing of benefits has been noted. *Sativa* is indicated for swelling of the nose or prostate, while *indica* is recommended for problems like sudden memory loss and ravenous overeating.

A prominent homeopath who died in 1929, William Boericke, M.D., wrote extensively about the use of cannabis in his work, *Homeopathic Materia Medica*. He divided his discussion between the properties of the tropical *Cannabis indica* and its resin and those of *Cannabis sativa,* or European hemp, and based his report on the experiments and observations of Dr. Albert Schneider. The result was one of the most comprehensive listings of subjective symptoms for which cannabis was considered helpful. What makes his research particularly valuable is the fact that it was undertaken in an era when cannabis was legal and research was not subject to political bias or legal penalties. Boericke made his general observations of the differences between *Cannabis indica* and *Cannabis sativa*. He collected subjective observations made after people ingested extremely heavy one-dram ($^1/_8$-oz.) doses of mother tincture.[8] Their reactions to massive doses were considered likely indications for the therapeutic use of extremely dilute doses of cannabis tinctures. Boericke recorded that patient responses to high doses of resin featured remarkable hallucinations and imaginations, exaggerated notions of time and space, and feelings of extreme happiness and contentment. The patient enters a dual state, acting simultaneously as observer and participant. Boericke noted that the tincture made with the resin was soothing for many nervous disorders like epilepsy, dementia, delirium tremens, mania, tinnitus, and irritable reflexes, as well as for exophthalmic goiter and catalepsy. His observations of European hemp were that it helped with conditions of the urinary, sexual, and respiratory organs, stuttering, and eye pain caused by pressure behind the eyes, but no mental effects were observed.

GANJA: AN AYURVEDIC MEDICINE

Almost every culture throughout history has utilized entheogens, psychoactive plants that have religious significance. The resinous cannabis flower is among the best known of those plants. The heavily populated, tropical land of India is so heavily steeped in the cultural and spiritual use of resinous cannabis that its people won a cultural exception to the UN Single Convention Treaty on Narcotic Drugs. It allows them to continue to consume the plant known as *ganja*. It is no surprise, then, that cannabis has a prominent role in the region's medical practices as well.

To understand the therapeutic use of ganja in India, one must understand the socio-spiritual framework in which it is practiced. Ganja was always integrated into and accepted by the culture of India. The *Vedas* are ancient writings that serve as the foundation of Hindu civilization. The classical authors deliberately kept their works brief and cryptic. *Ayurveda* is a traditional system of health care that regards each person as a unique combination of mind, intellect, ego, and soul, as well as an organism of skin, flesh, blood, and bone. Many drugs, including cannabis, are prescribed to maintain positive health, and to prevent or cure psychic, somatic, and psychosomatic diseases. The fundamental principles of Ayurvedic systems often combine applied treatments with philosophy and religion. Before cannabis is consumed, for example, the traditional blessing "bom shankar" is spoken.

While it is not scientific to accept traditions as true without proper verification, it is equally unscientific to reject them simply because they are traditional or old. Many things which were once treated as myth are now recognized as scientific facts.[9] The circulation of blood described before 700 B.C. in *Susruta samhita* was considered a myth until Leonardo da Vinci mapped the circulatory system, and later William Harvey traced the actual flow of blood. The secretion and role of gastric juices in the digestive process was described in Vedic times by *Caraka samhita*, but was thought to be a myth until Pavlov's dog experiments. The use of inoculation against smallpox was just another myth until it was demonstrated by Edward Jenner. Skeptics still refuse to believe that this procedure was undertaken in classical India to prevent an epidemic. The description of plastic surgery in *Susruta samhita* would still be considered a myth, were it not for recent advances made by plastic surgeons of the West. The head transplantation in the *Vedas* will continue to be treated as myth, and rightly so, until it is adequately demonstrated in accordance with modern standards.

Like any traditional system of medicine, ayurveda has distinctive features. It emphasizes the promotion of positive health and the prevention of disease. Health is the basis by which we achieve the inner goals of the self. The prevention and treatment of diseases includes the drugs and therapies prescribed in the classics and administered by Ayurvedic physicians. Some of these medicines have bacteriostatic or bactericidal effects, but most of them do not aim to kill these disease-bearing organisms. After all, drugs that kill harmful organisms quite often have a similar effect on the patient's own body tissues. When given in a dose sufficient to kill an invading organism, pharmaceutical drugs can also harm or kill friendly organisms in the body, weaken healthy organs, and impair vital tissues in their normal functions. The end result is that allopathic medicines often produce toxic side effects, even while curing the disease.

According to Ayurveda, health is an affirmative concept that implies an excellence of the soul, the senses, and the mind. Although we try to minimize our exposure to them, we will never live in an absolutely germ-free environment. The alternative, then, is to develop the body's inner resistance to these outside organisms. No germs or bacteria can produce a disease in the human body unless the body's tissues are vulnerable enough to accept and support the growth and multiplication of disease. The tissues of a body that has been afflicted should be conditioned by drugs, diet, and other therapies to foster a healthy environment that is hostile toward these invaders. Therefore, the measures prescribed in these traditional systems aim to condition the body rather than simply destroy germs. They must improve the whole self.

Ayurvedic medicines are therefore developed as tonics that nourish and rejuvenate body tissues while they condition it to resist disease. As a result, in addition to being cured of the disease, the patient often receives beneficial side effects. With few exceptions, such as minerals and vitamins, modern drugs are meant for use exclusively by patients. Ayurvedic drugs, on the other hand, can safely be administered both to patients and to healthy individuals. They cure disease in patients, and simultaneously prevent disease and promote positive well-being in healthy people—without fear of negative effects.

Cannabis in Ancient Hindu Medical Texts

With this general basis for understanding Ayurveda, we return our attention to the topic of cannabis drugs, including bhanga, ganja, and charas.

Cannabis hemp was used in India from the very beginning for both its fiber and entheogenic effects. Ganja, like many other important medicinal plants, is said to have originated from the primordial nectar which arose during the churning of oceans. In the *Atharva Veda* a plant called bhanga is mentioned as one of the five sacred plants headed by soma.[10] Although Sayana interpreted it as *sana*, a type of wild grass, the philologist W. W. D. Whitney accepted bhanga to mean resinous cannabis. Most scholars agree with Whitney, because bhanga is classified with soma, which later is known for its rejuvenating properties. According to mythology, cannabis drugs had different colors in different ages.[11] Tantrika texts have divided this plant into four types, corresponding to the Hindu caste system.[12] Different *mantras*—brief, spiritual chants or hymns—have been developed for use with the different types of cannabis.[13]

Most of the systems advocated in ancient Indian scriptures are spiritual in nature. However, the *Yoga Sutra* mentions that certain medicines may help to overcome worldly miseries while attaining spiritual perfection.[14] Cannabis is not mentioned by name in the oldest scriptures, but subsequent followers have described the resinous cannabis plant as being one such medicine which maintains the mental process, and thereby relieves suffering.[15] The *Tantra Sastra* prescribes that certain drugs be consumed to regulate mental functions, cannabis among them.[16]

Bhanga was known as a substance to be consumed in powder form according to Katyayana, the fourth-century B.C. author of a codex of supplementary rules.[17] An in-depth description of this plant and its medicinal properties was presented in the tenth-century text, *Anandakanda*. After this, its medicinal properties are described in numerous works on Ayurveda, although a certain amount of scholarly interpretation is required to properly identify the various, often poetic references. For example, cannabis is commonly referred to as bhanga and *vijaya* (victory) in Ayurvedic texts, whereas its most common name is *samvid* in tantric texts. Some of the plant's Sanskrit synonyms indicate its physical form and structure. In mythology, the cannabis leaf is compared to a trisula of Shiva, which indicates that each leaf is composed of leaflets which are pointed at the end, and sharp and serrated along the edge. About forty-three synonyms have been attributed to the cannabis plant, and the etymology behind many of them was traced and explained by Bhagwan Dash.

According to an important text, cannabis drugs are beneficial for a great variety of people.[18] Its consumers have been divided into four broad categories:

- Priests, ascetics, fakirs, yogis, and sanyasis (to stimulate meditation and a spiritual mindset).
- Devotees of Shiva, Kali, Durga, Hanuman, and other gods (for ceremonies).
- People who perform hard physical labor, to relieve their pain and fatigue.
- Patients, to relieve their psychic, somatic, and psycho-somatic ailments.

In tantric texts, cannabis is divided into eight varieties based on the number of leaflets per leaf.[19] Physicians and scholars of ancient India were well aware of the plant's sexuality. It is specifically noted that it is the female plant that produces potent medicinal effects, gives pleasure to the mind, and causes "fainting" if consumed in excess.[20] The female plant is described as pungent in taste and smell. Adding female ganja to any other medicine is said to cause a synergistic action that enhances the effect of the other medication.

Ganja is consumed as an ingredient in various foods, such as *barfee, laddoo, sarabat* (sweet drink), and a chewy green honey candy called *ma'joun.* Raw cannabis is chewed, sometimes along with the stimulant betel leaf. And, finally, people smoke it through a *chillum*—a chimney-style pipe used by Sadhu monks. Cannabis is also prescribed and consumed in the following Ayurvedic forms: powdered *(curna),* lumped into a bolus *(modaka),* pressed into a tablet *(vatika),* used as a tincture *(leha* and *paka),* boiled with milk *(dugdhapaka),* and boiled in water to produce a decoction *(kvatha).*

Cannabis is seldom used alone for specific medical preparations. It is usually combined with a variety of other medicines to reduce its natural psychotropic effects or broaden its therapeutic applications. Bhagwan Dash lists fifty-one important formulations for cannabis drugs. Some of these recipes clearly designate which parts of the cannabis plant to use and how to prepare the drug with due respect, in addition to the general rules for such purposes.[21] For example, some formulas specify that the seed be used in combination with vegetable drugs, drugs of metallic and mineral origin, or animal products. Other formulas call for processing the raw plant matter (boiling with milk, water, etc.) before using it, or specify which type of container to use to store it, or at what intervals the patients should take it. Physicians keep track of the age of the material and how long their medicine should be used.

It is considered appropriate in Ayurveda for both healthy individuals and patients with acute conditions to consume cannabis. Healthy people consume it as an aphrodisiac and a rejuvenating agent. Patients use it to treat these major ailments: Sprue syndrome,[22] male and female sterility, impotence, diarrhea, indigestion, epilepsy, insanity, and colic pain. In addition, this medicine in combination with others is indicated in the treatment of at least thirty-two other ailments, many of which have a familiar ring to them: rheumatism, gastritis, anorexia, fistula, throat obstruction, nausea, fever, jaundice, bronchitis, consumption, obstinate skin diseases (including leprosy), torticolis, spleen disorder, delirium, obstinate urinary disorders (including diabetes), the common cold, sinus congestion, anemia, chronic rhinitis (runny nose), painful menstruation, tuberculosis, elephantitis, edema (dropsy), puerperal sepsis, asthma, morbid thirst, vomiting, gout, diseases of the nervous system, constipation, malaria fever, and liver disease.[23]

It must be noted that Ayurvedic scholars of India have also attributed certain injurious effects to excess use of cannabis drugs, and recommend taking precautions. Its root is described as poisonous in *Susruta samhita*.[24] Numerous medieval works also describe decoction of hemp root as a minor poison.

While the cannabis flower is not toxic in the sense of having a lethal dosage, it does sometimes have undesirable side effects if consumed to excess. To reduce this form of "toxicity" and to increase its therapeutic efficacy, the herb can be boiled or fried in cow's milk before it is consumed. *Anandakanda* gives a detailed description of the resin's effects that occur in human beings in nine successive stages, and of the characteristic features of body and mind of the individual during each of these stages. Various methods have been suggested to counteract the acute effects, including purgation, head bath with cold water, use of fragrant and cooling flowers and ornaments, intake of betel leaves with spices, intake of drinks prepared with sugar, milk, and ghee (clarified butter), and complete bed rest.

A simple recommendation is to take a pinch of powdered calamus root with one-fourth to one-half teaspoon of honey in the morning and evening. According to tradition, calamus aids the liver, works on the higher cerebral functions and brain tissue to help expand and bring clarity to the consciousness, and helps improve the memory. Adding a pinch of this powder to the smoking mix is said to neutralize many of the undesirable side effects of smoking cannabis, as well as other psychedelics. Unfortunately, calamus is currently under FDA restrictions: the agency has not recommended it for internal usage and actually considers it toxic. Nonetheless, calamus is one of the most renowned traditional herbs of Ayurveda and has been consumed for thousands of years.

Cannabis for Ayurvedic Rejuvenation

Special ritualized methods are prescribed in Ayurveda for cultivating, collecting, processing, and preserving cannabis for personal rejuvenation.[25] Once the female colas are mature, harvest the cannabis plant. Dry it in a clean place in mild sunlight and place it on a large sterile vessel. Crush the herb into a fine powder and keep it between two hot plates for seven successive days to fully dry and complete the curing process. Mix a liter of milk with a kilogram of sugar and boil to make a syrup. Add 400 g of cannabis powder and 50 g each of eight other medicinal plants, and mix thoroughly. After the mixture cools, add a half liter each of honey and ghee and mix well. Keep the preparation inside a heap of grain for one month, and every day recite the appropriate mantras. Next, remove the medicine from the grain and consume in five-gram doses. While doing so, reside in a closed-up house for three years, observing celibacy and eating only milk and rice. By doing this periodically, it is claimed that a person can live free of any disease or signs of old age for three hundred years, which is a lot of milk, rice, and celibacy. The text that offers this regimen also describes at least fifty other different cannabis drug preparations for the purposes of rejuvenation, aphrodisiac effect, and cure of several diseases. Luckily, not all of them are this restrictive.

In the Indian philosophy of *Samkhya*, human miseries are separated into three categories: those of internal origin, which include psycho-somatic ailments; those of external origin; and those of divine origin. Similarly, the mind has three aspects: tranquility, momentum, and inertia, and physical disorders are represented in one or the other of these latter three aspects. Everything that is available in the individual is also present throughout the universe. In order to overcome his own attributes, the patient must offer prayer to deities that have similar attributes, such as Shiva and Kali. Cannabis is one of many items which are offered in different forms to both Shiva and Kali, and their priests and devotees partake of it after the ceremony. Until the time of the *Mahabharata*, the social custom of taking mind-altering substances was not the least bit stigmatized. But in the epic story of Kaca and Devayani, Sukracarya made a

serious blunder due to his alcoholic intoxication, so he prohibited the use of alcohol for himself and all Brahmins.[26] Cannabis,
on the other hand, was never banned, and has found a safe
shelter among the tantrikas of the left wing, as well as the devotees of Shiva and Kali. During medieval times, its rediscovery as
a medicine swept across India.

There is no direct reference to smoked cannabis in ancient
Ayurveda. Only bhanga and ganja were consumed internally.
Bhanga, the weakest form, is consumed in most of the medicines and religious ceremonies. Ganja is consumed exclusively
by some sects of mendicants. The use of charas resin arose after
the medieval era. With religious and social approval, cannabis
has been used at a responsible level which is not harmful to the
human body or mind. Respectful use of cannabis within a framework of religion, philosophy, and science survives to this day in
India and thus has never been considered an antisocial act. That's
a lesson that America is just starting to learn.

INTEGRATING CANNABIS INTO TOTAL HEALTH CARE

Centuries of battling disease have left some researchers and
allopaths with an antagonistic attitude toward other approaches
to healing. Perhaps this rift is beginning to mend. It is common
in practice for allopaths to use a variety of techniques simultaneously. Physical therapy regimens are known to enhance the
benefits of other orthodox medical treatments. Exercise increases
vigor and energy levels, tones various body systems, and stimulates both physical and neurological responses. The Chinese have
long advocated using a combination of healing systems to increase the overall benefit of treatment. They call this practice
"walking on two legs." Experimentation with a variety of therapeutic combinations is always wise.

Cannabis works as allopathic medicine, at the same time allowing patients and doctors to step away from the modern com-

mercial focus and return to the principles of the Hippocratic oath. In this venerable affirmation of the healing profession, physicians pledge to work for the good of their patients; to do them no harm; to prescribe no deadly drugs; to give no advice that could cause death; and to keep all patients' medical information confidential. Cannabis is a discrete and gentle remedy that meets all these criteria.

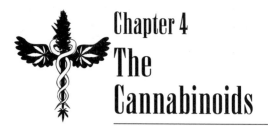

Chapter 4
The
Cannabinoids

The medical efficacy of THC is unquestionable, and THC pills are available internationally, yet the natural herb is a far superior medicine. The herb's resin contains at least sixty compounds. Many of them, such as cannabinol (CBN), cannabichromene (CBC), cannabidiol (CBD), and cannabigerol (CBG), have potential therapeutic value and can be isolated from both industrial hemp and resinous cannabis. These organic chemicals and their related analogs have been shown to have antimicrobial action.[1] Nonpsychoactive, they are generally not restricted by international regulations that prohibit cannabis and THC, nor are they being marketed commercially on any sizable economic scale.[2] The best available source is still natural cannabis.

Unfortunately, it's not easy to establish the cannabinoid profile of a given sample of herb. The process generally requires the use of gas chromatography, an accurate but expensive analysis procedure. Nonetheless, a patient can get a pretty good idea of what works and what doesn't and, given a range of cannabis over time, will begin to intuitively select and prepare cannabis with the organic profile that offers the most relief.

The apparent biochemical pathway of the major cannabinoids flows from olivetol to CBG, then to either CBC or CBD, and from there into THC. When a hydroxyl group (hydrogen plus oxygen) attaches to the molecule's terpene carbon, it signals the beginning of the molecule's transformation into CBN. Only the THC form is psychoactive; however, the hydroxyl stage, which also results when the liver metabolizes THC in digestion, is perhaps its most potent form.[3] This may explain why eating too much herb is more likely to cause unpleasant, but harmless, overdose effects.

Industrial hemp has been bred to maximize its fiber and minimize its THC content. International agreements recommend a level in the fiber strains of less than 0.3 percent THC.[4] Most varieties are even lower than this. Although soil, stress, plant density, and other environmental conditions also play a role in determining the ultimate THC level reached, cannabinoid levels achieved in the mature female buds are primarily caused by genetic factors. While selective breeding for high THC content was being conducted by many U.S. and Dutch marijuana growers, Europe's industrial hemp researchers bred for lower THC content. The Le Mans Institute in France has developed a CBG-dominant strain with 0.001 percent THC.[5] Recent evidence suggests that the French research team may have reached its long-standing objective of completely eliminating THC from this cultivar. Wild hemp growing in Riley County, Kansas, measured very low in THC content, below the European community's threshold for nonpsychoactive fiber hemp. The leaves and flowering tops ranged from 0.01–0.49 percent THC with a mean average of 0.14 percent. The unintended results were strains with high CBD content—as much as 1.7 percent.[6]

At the same time, in order to rationalize its acceptance of synthetic THC pills as a legal prescription drug while banning natural cannabis, the U.S. government claims that THC is the only medically active drug in cannabis. Many drug companies have tried unsuccessfully in their research to separate the medical from the psychoactive effects of THC.[7] Much research and development into the medical use of cannabis therefore concludes

Aspects of cannabis and some attributes

Variety or aspect	Common names	Major attributes
Cannabidiol	CBD	Provides multiple medical benefits, including movement disorders, anxiolitic, pain relief.
Cannabindon	Red oil	A concentrated liquid extract of cannabis resin. Can be added to food or smoking matter.
Indica	Afghani, Indica, stinky bud	A short, dense plant giving higher yield for indoor growing spaces. Strong aroma; effect has more "body," makes the patient feel more tired.
Industrial hemp	Bunk, dirtweed, ditchweed, hemp, rope, schwag	Farm crop used for hempseed, fiber, cellulose, hemi-cellulose, etc. to make commercial goods and medical supplies, like absorbent pads and fabrics for bandages. Produces negligible THC in temperate zones, but can be high in CBD content.
Leaf	Shake	Lower concentrations of THC. Higher proportion of CBD and other therapeutic compounds. Better for eating than for smoking.
Marijuana	Bhang, bud, dagga, ganja, grass, green cookies, greenies, herb, kif, kind, ma'joun, Mary Jane, pot, reefer, smoke, tea, weed, etc.	Preparations from resinous cannabis foliage with higher levels of active compounds, especially THC. The amount and ratio of cannabinoids gives various seed lines a particular characteristic and personality. Multiple medical benefits.

Aspects of cannabis and some attributes *(cont.)*

Variety or aspect	Common names	Major attributes
Resin	Charas, glands, hash, hashish, kif, polum (pollen), trichomes	Collected trichome glands in either loose or compacted form. High THC content.
Resinous bud or flower	Bud, chronic, cola, green bud, herb, kind bud, sticky bud	High THC content and ratio to CBD. Multiple medical benefits.
Sativa	Colombian, Mexican, Thai	Taller, leggier plant. Bigger yield per plant outdoors. Sweet aroma and taste. Effect is more cerebral, less tiring.
Seed	Hempseed	The cannabis fruit with many qualities of a grain kernel; seed oils contain essential fatty acids, proteins, and globulin within a rigid hull. Both internal and topical medical applications. All varieties of cannabis seed have similar characteristics. No THC, regardless of drug content in the foliage.
THC	Natural: tetrahydro-cannabinol Synthetic: dronabinol or Marinol	Psychoactive compound that is responsible for many neuro-logical and ocular benefits. The synthetic version is the only cannabinoid that can be legally prescribed.

Seasonal Change in THC/CBD Profiles of Industrial Hemp

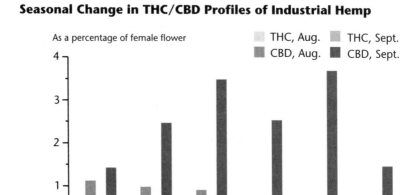

As a percentage of female flower

THC, Aug.   THC, Sept.
CBD, Aug.   CBD, Sept.

Seed Line   Fedora   Felina   Futura   Kompolti   Uniko   Kinai

with its offhand dismissal, due to its "unacceptable" (i.e., illegal) psychoactive effects.

Perhaps the most important nonpsychoactive compound in cannabis is CBD, which occurs in greater concentrations in industrial hemp.[8] A British study suggested that this could be an unexpected windfall for industrial hemp farmers: "Our results would suggest that cultivation of hemp plants rich in CBD and other phenolic substances would be useful not only as fiber producing plants but also for medicinal purposes in the treatment of certain inflammatory disorders."[9] Important research in Czechoslovakia and Brazil supports that contention.

Cannabidiol is a precursor compound in the organic pathway of the cannabinoids. It tends to maintain an inverse relationship with THC. Hence, industrial hemp is extremely low in THC, but high in CBD. In marijuana, THC is high, but CBD is low. In a third, intermediate type of cannabis, both THC and CBD levels are fairly high, which has a moderating influence on the psychoactive effect. A rodent study in Brazil found that CBD blocked some effects of THC in mice but potentiated others.[10] In a followup study on humans, CBD was found to block or suppress most of the demonstrated effects of THC, such as increased pulse rate, time distortion, and certain subjective reactions—particularly the anxiety response.[11] In 1982 researchers again verified that "the combination of the two cannabinoids significantly attenuated the anxiety and psychotomimetic effects" of THC.[12] In essence, CBD acts as a chemical buffer produced by the hemp plant to moderate the psychoactive cannabinoids.

The two major cannabinoids might be characterized as loving but competitive sisters. THC and CBD each try to outdo the other. Both are good-hearted nurses for sick and suffering humanity. Each have their own medicinal expertise and specialties. But, whereas THC likes to crack jokes and keep her patient smiling, CBD is quite serious and stops her sister's sense of humor in its tracks. That sibling rivalry makes the relationship between the two nurses as important to the patient's recovery as are the attentions of either one alone.

Aside from moderating the effects of THC, CBD is a potent allopathic medicine in its own right. Cannabidiol appears to be helpful for many medical conditions, with no adverse side effects. Among these are its activities as an anticonvulsant for epileptics, in easing dystonic movement disorders and symptoms of Huntington's disease, as an anti-inflammatory, as an aid to chronic insomnia, and as an antipsychotic.[13] Many of these conditions have long been known to respond well to natural cannabis, but are less successful when treated with THC alone. Furthermore, whereas the traditional use of cannabis as an analgesic, anti-asthmatic, and antirheumatic drug is well established, the role of CBD in soothing such conditions has only recently come to light. Cannabidiol was found to be a more effective anti-inflammatory agent than aspirin, as measured in the treatment of certain inflammatory disorders.[14] For research purposes, CBD is usually extracted from cannabis and orally ingested. As a means for self-medication, low-grade marijuana leaf can be smoked or eaten to ingest the CBD; even nonpsychoactive industrial hemp can be used—it just won't make you high.

Let's now review some direct applications of CBD that have been studied.

Dystonia is a painful condition marked by abnormal muscle rigidity, causing muscle spasms, unusually fixed postures, or strange movement patterns. It may affect a localized area of the body or it may be more generalized. The most common types of localized dystonia are painful neck spasm and an abnormal curvature of the spine caused by back injury. More generalized cases occur as a result of various neurological disorders, including Parkinson's disease and stroke. This problem can occur as a feature of schizophrenia or as a side effect of antipsychotic drugs. Cannabidiol was given to five patients who exhibited serious dystonic disorders. All five patients experienced a 20–50 percent improvement.[15]

Chorea is a neurological condition characterized by irregular, rapid, jerky movements or fidgets, usually affecting the face, limbs, and trunk. These involuntary movements occur at random intervals while awake, but not at all during sleep. This condition arises from disturbance of structures deep within the brain, especially the paired nerve-cell groups of the basal ganglia, or it can be a side effect of certain prescription drugs. Choreic movement is a consequence of diseases such as cerebral palsy, Sydenham's chorea, and Huntington's disease. Three patients with Huntington's disease, who had not been responsive to conventional therapy with neuroleptics, were given CBD.[16] After the second week, the frequency and intensity of choreic movement had declined in each of them by 20 to 40 percent. Except for transient, mild hypotension, no side effects were recorded.

Epilepsy is a convulsive condition that results from abnormal electrical activities in the brain and can be caused by a number of diseases and injuries, particularly head trauma. Episodic seizures occur spontaneously or may be triggered by external stimuli, such as flashing lights. Use of cannabis has proven helpful in many cases, but in a few cases it has also been suspected of triggering episodes. These rare incidents seem to have involved high-THC varieties. In an effort to identify its role in the sei-zure-suppression mechanism, eight epileptic patients in Brazil were given CBD.[17] Only one remained unchanged. Four of them remained free of convulsions for the entire duration of the treat-ment, and three had significant reductions in the frequency and intensity of seizures. No serious side effects were found, and the potential of CBD as an anti-epileptic drug was discussed in a published report. Another significant finding was the compound's possible role in potentiating the effects of other drugs. This synergy is important, because complex partial sei-zures involving secondary generalization patterns are difficult to treat with currently allowed drugs.

Sleep is the mechanism that allows the human constitution to rest, recuperate, and revive itself. The psyche dreams its sub-lime dreams and the body mends its cellular tissues. Insomnia is a physically exhausting condition that renders patients unable to sleep either soundly enough or long enough to fully rest or adequately replenish their energy. It can result from nervous conditions, disease, or metabolism, or as a side effect of various pharmaceutical drugs. Certain kinds of marijuana, especially leaf, have a reputation for making the consumer feel tired. Its use as a hypnotic sedative to treat insomnia has been documented for centuries. In a controlled study, fifteen insomniacs in Brazil were given 160 mg each of extracted CBD over a five-week period in the 1980s. Two-thirds of them slept for seven hours or more per night during the study after taking CBD. "Most subjects had few interruptions and reported having a good night's sleep."[18]

Since CBD reduces the psychological effects of THC, re-searchers are also looking into using it to help with a variety of psychological disorders. Another Brazilian study investigated the compound's possible antipsychotic activity on animal models being used to research potential antipsychotic drugs.[19] Canna-bidiol compared favorably with haloperidol as an antipsychotic. This raises interesting possibilities for human research.

Tourette's syndrome (TS) is a lifelong neurological condition that usually begins in childhood with repetitive grimaces and facial tics, and occasionally tics in the limbs and trunk. At first, these dyskinetic movements are often interpreted as misbehavior on the part of the child. As the disease progresses, involuntary barks, grunts or other noises may appear. In about half the cases, the sufferer has episodes of *coprolalia*, involuntary outbursts of foul language. Once diagnosed, it is usually treated with antipsychotic drugs, such as haloperidol. However, three TS patients who had been only partially helped by conventional drugs noted a significant improvement of symptoms after smoking cannabis.[20] This benefit may be related to CBD's anxiety-reducing properties, although a more specific anti-dyskinetic effect cannot be excluded.

Don't expect to keep marijuana illegal and just use industrial hemp as a medicine, however. For all the benefits we find ascribed to CBD, remember that THC is so much more powerful a medicine that the federal government claims it is the only medicinal compound in the plant. The truth is that the various cannabinoids potentiate and moderate one another's effects and work best in their natural combinations.

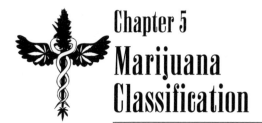

Chapter 5
Marijuana
Classification

The vast amount of pharmaceutical information that is now available can be managed only if drugs are put into classes or categories. The same properties that make a therapeutic agent useful may also make for an enticing social drug, and it is not surprising that most social drugs fit into known categories. We need to establish where cannabis stands in the overall scheme of pharmacology to better understand its potential.

The law lists marijuana as a hallucinogen, and any number of groups and individuals seek to confuse the discussion by referring to cannabis as a "mild hallucinogen." This label was merely a matter of convenience for the federal DEA when it implemented the Controlled Substance Act so it would not have to create a separate category for cannabis.[1]

In extremely large doses, cannabis extracts and analogs bear many similarities to the psychedelics (though the same could be said of nutmeg and many other common substances). Marked distortion of auditory and visual perception, hallucinations, and depersonalization have been described by researchers. The peculiar wave-like experience of effects is also similar for both types of drugs but, as a psychotomimetic, LSD is 160 times more potent than THC.[2]

THC/CBD Profiles of Psychoactive Cannabis

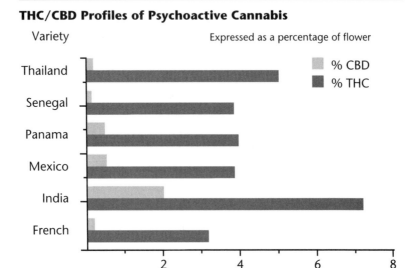

There are numerous other important differences between cannabis and the strong hallucinogens. The subjective effects of the two drugs are readily distinguished by consumers. The psychoactive effects of even large doses of marijuana are milder and more easily controlled than those of LSD. Increased pulse rate and conjunctival reddening are common for cannabis but not for LSD or mescaline,[3] while THC, even at high doses (70 mg), appears to lack the major effects of biochemical and clinical measures of stress found with the psychotomimetics.[4] Tolerance is not appreciable for cannabis at the usual doses, but it occurs very rapidly with psychotomimetics; moreover, there is no cross-tolerance in man between THC and LSD.[5] Acute changes in brain wave patterns characteristic of LSD are absent with marijuana.[6] Cannabis resination ends in sedation and sleep while restlessness is characteristic of true hallucinogens.

CANNABIS COMPARED TO ALCOHOL

Alcoholic beverages are the preferred social drug of Americans, with cannabis a distant second in total user population. In low doses, the effects of marijuana and ethyl alcohol are similar, though the margin of safety for THC is far greater than that for alcohol.[7] Both produce an initial excited phase, followed by a later sedated one. Both are commonly used as euphoriants, relaxants, and intoxicants. At low doses, subjects have difficulty differentiating the effects of alcohol or marijuana from a smoked placebo that looks, smells, and tastes like marijuana. This respose diminishes, however, as the dosage increases.[8] In large doses, alcohol acts as a general anesthetic by producing a primary and continuous depression of the central nervous system. Experiments have shown that alcohol slows brain wave rhythms and decreases mental and physical performance, but does not alter sensory perceptions.[9] Cannabis, on the other hand, affects the consumer's perception but has negligible effect on brain waves.

A study compared the effects of marijuana extract (27–37 mg THC) with 95 percent ethyl alcohol (50–60 gm dose), in terms of mood and mental function. Neither changed blood sugar level but alcohol decreased free fatty acid level. Both produced euphoria, sleepiness, and decreased activity and performance on psychometric tests. Marijuana led to moderate overestimation of time while alcohol produced grossly exaggerated underestimation. Hunger and food consumption were increased by marijuana and decreased by alcohol.[10] Another study compared the effect of smoked marijuana (5–10 mg THC) with a sub-intoxicating level of alcohol (equivalent to three bottles of beer for a 150-pound man). This was the threshold level that resulted in diminished performance in a previous study with these tests, about 0.08 percent blood alcohol content. Performance of motor and mental function tests was undertaken while the subject was distracted by delayed auditory feedback. The study concluded that some performance decrease was produced by marijuana and that the combination of alcohol and marijuana generally led to a poorer performance than either drug alone.[11]

Alcoholic beverages must be ingested in grams rather than milligrams, and they provide empty calories that can take the place of healthy food, resulting in a loss of protein and vitamins, and in some people a thiamin deficiency that can lead to atrophy of the brain. Alcohol also has direct toxic effects on the liver, upper respiratory tracts, and brain. Its destructive nature, heavy commercial promotion, and the ease with which disinhibition can be reached have made alcohol responsible for massive social and criminal problems. Marijuana, on the other hand, is not associated with any of alcohol's serious physical or sociological problems.

SEDATIVE EFFECTS OF CANNABIS

A very large number of drugs can be listed in the categories of *anxiolytics, sedatives, hypnotics,* and *general anesthetics.* The differences between various sedatives are largely matters of the onset and duration of action. It is important, therefore, to study the drug over a range of doses, because the effects that appear at any one dose level may mislead. Marijuana is a drug which is pharmacologically similar to sedatives, but it does not necessarily follow that these sedative effects are induced regularly, or even at all, as marijuana is used socially in our culture. However, a significant relationship has been established through quantitative animal experiments and controlled clinical observations.

Both sedatives and marijuana follow a distinct progression of effects at doses of increasing size. Stage 1, small analgesic doses, causes the subject to experience relief of anxiety or a positively good feeling, and possibly some drowsiness. As dosage increases, psychomotor performance, concentration, and short-term memory become progressively impaired. Stage 2 begins with the appearance of excitement and ends with the loss of consciousness. In between, the highest cortical centers are increasingly depressed, and lower centers and more primitive behaviors are released from the inhibition that ordinarily controls them from above. Stage 3, the knocked-out level of surgical anesthesia, is easy to reach with cannabis in laboratory animals but almost unattainable in humans. Stage 4, medullary paralysis, is difficult to achieve in animals and has never been demonstrated in humans.

Frequent consumers of marijuana show reverse tolerance; they achieve higher plasma levels after a test dose and excrete the dose over a longer period than do infrequent consumers.[12] However, the abrupt substitution of a placebo after an extended period of receiving extreme doses of THC, not marijuana, led one subject to exhibit signs of hyperexcitability or stimulation—low-level withdrawal symptoms.[13] That response indicates a potential for some minor tolerance to develop with extremely heavy cannabis use.

OVERALL COMPARISON

Resinous cannabis involves many subtleties and cannot be accurately classified with a uniform dose level. Psychotomimetic effects are possible at high oral doses, particularly using pure THC or concentrated resin extracts, but these doses are rarely attained or sought after by consumers. An acute psychoactive agent, cannabis resembles alcohol qualitatively but does not produce the same gross effects on the central nervous system, general physiology, and behavior.

Cannabis is pharmacologically unique and distinct from the hallucinogens, opiates, barbiturates, and amphetamines. It may be closer to the sedatives than any other readily identifiable classification of drugs. In small doses, stimulation is followed by sedation. Because of significant differences between cannabis and even the sedatives, cannabis should comprise its own class of substance, and should be grandfathered into the pharmacopoeia as a traditional medicinal herb.

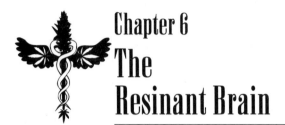

Chapter 6
The Resinant Brain

Whereas Ayurvedic healers consider the human soul as a factor in maintaining good health, Western physicians prefer to focus on the human brain. That brain is about 5 percent fat, most of which is located along the surface membranes, where much of our mental activities occur. Cannabinoids are fat soluble. When a compound attaches to a cell membrane, it changes the activity within the membrane, which in turn alters the way the cell processes information. The modified data is then dispatched throughout the nervous system. Because cannabis also goes directly to the organs, it can simultaneously reduce symptoms in multiple parts of the body in a variety of subtle but effective ways.

Cannabinoids have not been found to harm brain cells or nerve tissue. Dr. Igor Grant compared twenty-nine pairs of cannabis smokers and non-smokers in the 1970s and concluded that "A battery of the most sensitive neuro-psychological tests now available could demonstrate essentially no differences between moderate users and non-users of marijuana." Subsequent research has continued to find no significant differences between the control population and marijuana users, even in the case of heavy and very heavy users.[1]

In the fall of 1988, a group of St. Louis University Medical School researchers announced their discovery of a receptor site on the membrane of mouse nerve cells.[2] THC, considered the most powerful compound in cannabis resin, was found to attach to the brain at these points. Two years after this cannabinoid-specific protein receptor was reported, a group at the National Institute of Mental Health pinpointed the DNA that encodes the same receptor in rats. It is now known that people have the THC receptor, too. In the human brain, these cannabinoid-receptors are clustered in several areas. The cerebral cortex, the primary area, is also the home of higher thinking, perception, emotions, and cognition. Other clusters appear in the hippocampus, the section of the brain associated with memory; the cerebellum and striatum, which are associated with movement; and the basal ganglia, an area involved in movement control and coordination.

This produces the psychoactive effect of cannabis, as well as its amazingly broad effect on neuralgic and musculoskeletal functions throughout the human body. Research at the National Institute of Mental Health suggests that the arrangement of these receptor sites indicates that THC analogs and antagonists might eventually serve to ease symptoms of movement disorders like the tremors of Parkinson's disease and Huntington's chorea.[3] Cannabinoids could also possibly affect the transfer of data between the three memory centers: immediate, short-term, and long-term. The limbic system of the brain surrounds the upper stem and includes the hippocampus. Long-term memory is thought to reside in the mid-brain and cerebral cortex. Short-term memory is associated with the upper brain stem. Immediate memory is a function of the cortex. The possibility of using cannabis to treat memory disorders like Alzheimer's has yet to be adequately explored.

Once the human brain's receptors were identified, researchers extrapolated that there must be a natural, internal chemical that connected to the cannabinoid-receptor and sent

Important Compounds in Cannabis

Olivetol

Cannaflavon

CBG
Cannabigerol

CBD
Cannabidiol

THC
Tetrahydrocannabinol

CBN
Cannabinol

biochemical signals cascading through the nerve cell to produce its effect.

ANANDAMIDE

In 1992 William Devane and Raphael Mechoulam of Hebrew University identified the natural brain molecule that binds to the cannabinoid receptor. Mechoulam, famous for his discovery of delta-9-THC in the 1960s, pursued a strategy of investigating other chemicals that, like THC, are fat soluble. By separating these substances from those that are water soluble, his group extracted from pig brain an oily, hairpin-shaped chemical substance that attached to the cannabinoid receptor. They called it *anandamide*, from the Sanskrit word *ananda*, for "eternal bliss." A small sample was sent to Roger Pertwee, a pharmacologist at Aberdeen University, who had devised a sensitive test for cannabinoids that monitored a substance's ability to stop muscle-twitching in mouse tissue, when dropped on certain nerves. Pertwee ran his tests on Mechoulam's experimental substance. "We didn't know what it was—just that it was a greasy substance." But the anandamide depressed the twitch just like THC, and that December the results were published in the journal *Science*. The results of follow-up studies showed that anandamide acted like a very precise key that would lock only onto cells containing the receptor. Once anandamide attached to the cells, it triggered biochemical changes similar to those of THC and related chemicals. Not only did the substance fit the same lock as THC, it also seemed to open similar neurological doors.

The discovery of this lipid-soluble fatty acid was hailed as a major breakthrough. Researchers are still trying to identify which membranes cause the psychoactive effects of resinous cannabis, in efforts to formulate new compounds that attach to the anandamide molecule and lock onto those specific sites. That could presumably allow the compounds to bond with the brain and block the effect of the THC while having their own distinct effect. Scientists hope that such a substitute will also be useful for chemically triggering therapeutic activity within the brain to mimic or expand upon the health benefits of cannabis.

Two additional natural anandamides have recently been found. According to Mechoulam, all three known anandamides bind to the same receptor. They are actually a family of closely related compounds, which is common with other fatty acid derivatives in the body, such as prostaglandin and the leukotriens. The anandamides seem to have the same biological activity, and research is ongoing as to possible differences. When anandamides are injected into the brain, the concentration of cortical steroids goes up. There are indications that the steroids themselves may act on the cannabinoid receptor, presumably bringing down its activity.

While the most famous receptors to be found are in the brain, a peripheral receptor has been found in the spleen. Mechoulam suggests that this receptor may have something to do with the immune system.[4] There is also a receptor in the testes. A paper in the proceedings of the National Academy of Sciences indicates that both THC and anandamide affect the activation of the sperm before it fertilizes the egg, but the relevancy of that information has not been established. As yet, no data have identified any harmful consequences.

IMPROVING NEUROLOGICAL RESPONSIVENESS

Cannabis can ease the neurological and muscle problems associated with diseases such as multiple sclerosis (MS).[5] Some 350,000 people in the United States are estimated to have MS. Nationally, 8000 new cases are reported each year. The condition occurs more frequently in women, and most cases are diagnosed between the ages of thirty and fifty. In progressive stages, it interferes with the patient's ability to walk, stand, or control limbs and fingers. Cannabis has been demonstrated, in measured response laboratory studies, to relieve MS-related cramps, spasticity, and ataxia.[6] This helps individuals regain control over their limbs and allows them to function in routine physical activities that many of us take for granted, such as being able to walk with relative ease and comfort.

These neurological benefits apparently extend to amputees who experience the phantom limb effect, as well as to persons with certain rare abnormalities, such as multiple congenital cartilaginous exostosis and nail-patella syndrome. In such cases, cannabis and its extracts relieve pain and depression, serve as antispasmatics, and perform a variety of other functions.[7] Cannabis has also been used to quiet the tremors in *paralysis agitans*, and to bring great relief in cases of spasm of the bladder due to cystitis or nervousness.[8]

Resinous cannabis has been documented to help in controlling spasticity caused by spinal cord injury.[9] Richard is a Texas entrepreneur who knows this from personal experience. He is a paraplegic who gets around using a wheel chair, but has muscle spasms in his lower limbs. Richard began to smoke cannabis soon after the accident to cope with his depression, and quickly realized that it also helped control his spasms. When he began to grow his own herb, his attitude improved greatly, and his dry sense of humor returned. Facing his situation with renewed courage and optimism, he determined to be as self-sufficient as possible and learned how to drive a car by hand. Richard opened a store to sell industrial hemp products alongside cannabis smoking accessories, and later formed a buyers club to provide medicine for a few other patients. His use of cannabis enables Richard to continue to be a contributing member of society.

Cannabis can also suppress epileptic seizures and ease recovery after an episode. THC has been found to have a synergistic effect with diphenylhydantoin and Phenobarbital in reducing the frequency, length, and severity of seizures.[10] Still, it must be noted that in some cases cannabis use may have triggered epileptic episodes, so caution should always be exercised in this regard. Valerie Corral is a California woman who suffered serious injuries and head trauma in an automobile accident. Afterwards, she began to experience *gran mal* epileptic seizures. Her systematic use of cannabis enabled her to do three things: avert seizures before they occurred, mitigate the degree and intensity of any seizures that did occur, and speed up the recovery process after a seizure. Since beginning this therapy, her condition has been stable for years. Valerie still has cortex trauma and ongoing neurological problems, but she has learned to recognize the onset of a *gran mal* seizure as being preceded by the appearance of visual auras around objects. Smoking cannabis reduces the auras and stops her attacks from occurring. Although she still gets the auras, Valerie has been able to avoid having any major seizures for many years. She has been arrested on several occasions for her medical use of cannabis, and has repeatedly had the privacy of her home violated. One arrest went to trial in Santa Cruz. Her testimony, along with that of her family, her doctors, and other medical experts, convinced the jurors that Valerie needs to use cannabis and is not a threat to society, so she was acquitted. She and her husband Michael struggle to maintain a stoical attitude toward her situation, and have become caregivers who operate a medical marijuana growers' cooperative for patients. They were active in the campaign for the California Medical Marijuana Initiative, Proposition 215, and received recognition as a nonprofit health-care provider shortly after its passage in 1996.

PAIN CONTROL AND MIGRAINE HEADACHE

Cannabis can be particularly valuable for the relief of neuralgia—pain that is caused by nerve disturbance.[11] Pain reduction is frequently cited in the medical literature, as well as by patients themselves, as being a primary reason for cannabis use. Cannabis is also useful in menopausal headaches, and if these headaches are associated with constipation and anemia, iron and aloe have been recommended to be given simultaneously.[12] To relieve toothache, peasant farmers in Poland, Russia, and Lithuania commonly inhaled the vapors of smoldering seeding tops of hemp plants that were thrown onto hot stones.[13]

This is how one patient explained her experience using cannabis both to control chronic pain and to reduce her use of pharmaceuticals. "I have CFIDS and kidney disease with several symptoms of lupus. I have been in severe pain over the past several years. I was taking narcotic pain killers for quite some time. I got side effects from most of the pain killers, and a lot of them were not good for my kidneys. Recently I began to smoke marijuana. Since I began doing this, I feel great! I have motivation. I exercise. I am in a good mood. I am not complaining that I do not feel well. . . . All I know is I got my life back. This is so much safer than the other drugs. My pharmacy bill has gone down quite a bit."

Migraine affects 10 percent of the population, three times more women than men. It is a severe headache lasting hours or days, frequently accompanied by blurred vision, nausea, and vomiting. Migraine may strike children, in fact 60 percent of sufferers have their first attack before age twenty. An attack in a susceptible person can be triggered by stress, menstruation, foods (chocolate, dairy, red wine, citrus, and fried foods are famous culprits), or overstimulation of the senses (bright lights, loud noise). Migraine begins as a slowly developing, throbbing pain, especially on one side of the head, accompanied by other symptoms. The intensity often recedes after vomiting. The best treatment is for the sufferer to keep track of what circumstance or activity preceded the attack, and avoid this trigger. Once an attack is underway, however, the treatment is to sleep in a dark room and combine an analgesic with an antiemetic. Cannabis naturally combines these last two features, and it may help the patient sleep, as well. Before the introduction of antipyrine and its congeners, tincture of *gelsemium* (an extract from the yellow jasmine plant) taken with tincture or extract of cannabis was our best remedy for the treatment of migraine.[14] Further attacks can be prevented by the use of small amounts of cannabis during the intervals. Patient case histories and the limited amount of research done with CBD indicate that using leaf may be more effective than bud for treating migraine.

Carol lives in the Emerald Triangle section of Northern California and manufactures various hempseed oil products, such as soaps and lip balm. She also wrote one of the first modern hempseed cookbooks. She suffers from various allergies and first experienced a migraine at the age of fourteen. "The sparkling, flickering visual effects, which were curious at first, consumed me so that I could not see the blackboard." She left the classroom and vomited for several hours before being taken home for the day. The attacks went on for years, but were not diagnosed as migraine until college. She was then prescribed various opiate medications, and later a number of barbiturates, but she found that they made her lightheaded, sleepy, and disoriented, and otherwise interfered with her normal functioning. Her husband mentioned that he had heard that marijuana might help. To her amazement, after only one or two puffs and a short rest, the nausea and headache went away. "As soon as I noticed flickering visuals that forewarned me of an approaching migraine, I could take a little cannabis and a short nap." That stopped the migraine from taking hold, and she could resume her normal activities within half an hour. When her older daughters began to experience migraine, she let them try cannabis, too, with impressive results.

MODERATING PSYCHOLOGICAL EFFECTS

Applied research has demonstrated several psychological benefits of cannabis as a form of therapy. As mentioned earlier, psychotherapy was among the first Western uses of cannabis drugs, as employed by French military physicians in Egypt. In an 1897 review of hashish in the *British Medical Journal*, a physician reported that, "from a frequent observation of hemp, both subjective and objective, I can affirm that it is soothing and stimulating, being when inhaled a specially valuable cerebral stimulant. I believe it to be an exceedingly useful therapeutic agent, one not likely to lead to abuse, and producing in proper dosage no untoward after-effects."[15]

The euphoriant effect of cannabis is particularly beneficial for depression patients, but its resin also moderates the extreme mood swings experienced by manic depressives. This antidepressant effect was first demonstrated under modern clinical conditions by researchers who contributed to the LaGuardia report in 1942.[16] Their study also verified the value of cannabis in treating appetite loss and opiate addiction. A few years later, a British study again showed the medical utility of cannabis in treating depression.[17] Out of fifty depression patients who received large doses of cannabis extract, thirty-six showed improvement. Follow-up studies were less successful, whether due to drug, dosage, setting, or design. In most cases, much lower doses were given than those used in the British study. In the most recent trial, in 1973, the researchers themselves noted that "the relatively brief duration of the trial (one week) must be kept in mind, since standard antidepressants require two to three weeks to produce clinical improvement."[18] With no subsequent research having been done in this regard, we must look to a patient's case history as a way to gauge the efficacy of cannabis.

The other side of depression is the wildly energized experience of mania, and for people who have both conditions, life is a see-saw of emotional and physical ups and downs. A Virginia woman described her experience using cannabis to control her manic depression like this. "Suppose I am in a fit of manic rage—the most destructive behavior of all. A few puffs of this herb, and I can be calm. My husband and I have both noticed this; it is quite dramatic. One minute out of control in a mad rage over a meaningless detail, seemingly in need of a strait jacket, and somewhere, deep in my mind, asking myself why this is happening and why I can't get a handle on my own emotions. Then, within a few minutes, the time it takes to smoke a few pinches—why, I could even, after a round of apologies, laugh at myself! But this herb is illegal, and I have a strong desire to abide by the law. . . . I took lithium for six months and experienced several adverse side effects—shaking, skin rashes, and loss of control over my speech. . . . The combination of lithium side effects and increased manic-depressive symptoms drove me back to the use of cannabis. . . . Cannabis does not cure my condition, and over the years it has probably continued to worsen. But with judicious use of this medicine, my life is fine. I can control things with this drug. . . . Often I do not experience a 'high' at all, just a return to normal."[19] This moderating function of cannabis is critical for her to maintain her stability. Her situation has also responded to the use of THC pills, although she prefers the natural herb.

When a patient is prescribed a series of interactive medications to treat a condition, cannabis may actually serve the same function as some pharmaceutical drugs, such as Valium, or it may help mitigate some of the other drugs' side effects. The herb can also provide a pleasant distraction from traumatic or distressing life situations, as was noted among U.S. troops in Vietnam.

The federal government has done a number of clandestine research projects in New Mexico and elsewhere using Vietnam veterans suffering from Posttraumatic Stress Disorder (PTSD), with significant findings that have not yet been made readily available. Many veterans who first experienced cannabis in Southeast Asia have found it to be quite useful in dealing with the flashbacks and sudden fits of anger, anxiety, and depression that are associated with the disorder. Curiously enough, veterans of the 1991 Persian Gulf War also report that the effects of Gulf War Syndrome appear to be mitigated by the use of cannabis. Recent evidence indicates that these troops were exposed to doses of nerve gas a number of times during the conflict. The exact nature of the neurological benefits of cannabis in both these situations may not be properly understood until the government ends its ongoing cover-up of what really happened to these veterans.

The U.S. Department of Veterans Affairs conducted a secret study of marijuana use among veterans suffering from PTSD, to determine the reasons for marijuana use and how side effects from marijuana differs between different diagnostic categories of psychiatric patients. Preliminary data suggest both similarities and differences in why mental health patients use it and what side effects they experience. Many patients from all diagnostic groups reported use of marijuana to help relax and to socialize. The PTSD group more often used marijuana to help with sleep, decrease nightmares, prevent bad memories of the past, and improve self-esteem. Bipolar patients tended to use marijuana to stabilize their mood. Depressed patients often reported use for "fun." Schizophrenics reported more unpleasant side effects than did patients with other diagnoses.[20]

Ingesting a minute, homeopathic dose of cannabis tincture can reduce or eliminate the pathological ringing sound in the ears known as *tinnitus*. Some anecdotal reports indicate that a puff or two of cannabis can bring relief, as well. It is suggested that the micro-dose neurologically inoculates the nervous system against having hallucinations, thereby immunizing it against responding to internally generated sounds. Cannabis was popularly used in the 1960s and 1970s to help people who were experiencing discomfort, anxiety, and overwhelming hallucinogenic effects from taking LSD. Particularly for those who had used cannabis before, the herb seemed to reduce the visual brilliance of the experience, lower overall stress and restore a level of familiarity that allowed the subject to cope with their mental situation a little better. Conversely, it has also been smoked near the end of an LSD experience to allow the subject to extend their experience or trigger a new level of psychedelic thought and visual stimulation.

Although cannabis and its extracts can be useful for patients suffering from psychosis,[21] its use should be approached with a great deal of caution and in a closely monitored setting. High doses of THC can cause anxiety, which could potentially trigger or aggravate a psychotic episode in an at-risk personality. This is particularly true if high doses of pure THC are used without any buffers to reduce anxiety. Fortunately, natural cannabis resin produces lower concentrations of THC, and mixes in the anxiolitic compound CBD. Federal Bureau of Narcotics psychiatrist Dr. Walter Bromberg noted in 1938 that "The patient who is developing a functional psychosis strives in the incipient stage to overcome the unconsciously perceived difficulties. In this sense [cannabis] usage represents a healthy reactive tendency, even though the mechanism may be unknown to the patient."[22] In the 1990s, Harvard Psychiatrist Dr. Lester Grinspoon has had success prescribing THC pills for depressive and manic-depressive patients.[23] Unfortunately, the pills do not contain CBD. Hence, for a more balanced effect, a patient is better off using cannabis flowers.

A major advantage of cannabis over many other mood-altering drugs is that the patient remains fully functional and in control. Cannabis smokers retain their mental faculties, personal responsibility, and a relatively high degree of mental clarity. They remain aware of their physical pains and problems, but also feel a sense of detachment that helps them keep things in proportion. This perspective, along with the herb's pain-relieving effects, has played a profound role in helping terminal patients face their impending deaths with courage and dignity. The nineteenth-century physician William O'Shaughnessy poetically described this sublime and soothing effect as enabling the physician "to strew the path to the tomb with flowers."

Lest I begin to sound too enthusiastic, however, it should be noted that anecdotal evidence indicates that overuse of cannabis has, in some cases, led people to feel distracted, uncomfortable, lacking in motivation, unclear in their thinking, or even somewhat dependent on using cannabis as a way to cope with everyday life. Adolescents and addictive personalities are particularly at risk in this regard. Whenever anything gets in the way of normal functioning, its use should be reevaluated and modified or discarded.

In any case, marijuana is not physically addictive. Its use does not automatically lead to escalated dosages, physical dependence, and delirium or painful withdrawal. To the contrary, familiarity usually leads to increased sensitivity and the use of lower dosages, while most regular users find a comfortable level of usage—perhaps saving it for weekends or after work—and maintain that pattern for years on end. For the vast majority of consumers, ending their use of cannabis is simply a matter of willpower.

Various studies have also shown cannabis to be useful in drug abuse diversion, including drug substitution and alcohol withdrawal.[24] Cannabis has been used to mitigate withdrawal symptoms from alcohol and heroin in human populations.[25] A similar benefit has been demonstrated in animal models. A number of people have described wild, alcoholic indulgences in their teen years and early adulthood, and credited their discovery of the benefits of smoking cannabis for having diverted them from a life of recklessness and physical deterioration. All of these individuals have family histories of alcohol abuse. Several people have also reported that they use cannabis to help them deal with the physical toll that resulted from years of heavy drinking, and also use the herb to satisfy their social cravings and keep them from relapsing into alcoholism.

In each of their circumstances, although they use more cannabis than they might wish, the patients indicate that any problems caused pale in comparison to the addictions, physical deterioration, and social harm from which this healing herb has saved them.

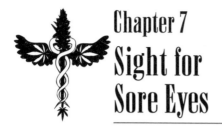

Chapter 7
Sight for
Sore Eyes

The eyes are a sensory extension of the brain, organic light detectors through which we gather visual data and convert it into neurological impulses. More poetically, the eyes have been described as windows to the soul. Cannabis can help those windows remain clear.[1]

Inner ocular pressure (IOP) has nothing to do with blood pressure. It has to do with the eye's regulation of a watery fluid called *aqueous humor*. This fluid normally circulates through the eye in a flow that drains away through tiny funnels along the rim of the iris, where it meets the cornea. The blockage of these funnels has potentially disastrous consequences. Glaucoma is a condition which interferes with the eyes' normal release mechanisms and raises the IOP up to dangerous levels. It is one of the nation's leading causes of blindness. In glaucoma, the angle at the opening of those tiny funnels causes them to close up, resulting in a backup of aqueous fluids. This is somewhat analogous to closing the floodgates on a dam in a river to produce a lake. The problem is, you don't want those valves closed, because the eye is too fragile to withstand the resulting pressure. The buildup of pressure squeezes the sensitive ocular nerves and blocks the flow of visual data, causing cumulative deterioration. The optical nerves do not normally repair themselves once tissue has been damaged, so each episode results in a progressive loss of vision. The result is a gradual loss of peripheral vision and the development of tunnel vision, in which the patient is steadily limited to an ever-shrinking field of sight. Unless the eye pressure is brought down to a safe level, the patient will go blind. Many sufferers of glaucoma who face sensory deprivation find fast relief in the cannabis flower's ability to lower the fluid pressure inside the eyeball itself.

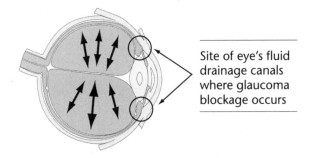

Site of eye's fluid drainage canals where glaucoma blockage occurs

Glaucoma accounts for 15 percent of blindness. In the United States alone, three to four million people have this disease and are at risk of serious loss of sight, particularly senior citizens. About 6 percent of Americans over the age of sixty-five encounter the condition. One out of fifty persons under the age of thirty-five has suspiciously high pressure that could warrant further investigation. Few daily marijuana smokers are among them, because regular use of the herb helps hold down the pressure and prevent this painful process. Cannabis drugs have been shown to reduce IOP in lab animals as well as, or better than, conventional pharmaceutical drugs, with fewer or no medical side effects.[2] In recent years, THC and other derivatives have also successfully been extracted for eye drops, but cannabis works without directly acting on the glaucomatous process.[3] Orthodox medical strategies seek to open up those drainage ducts either by chemistry or by surgery. Cannabis uses a different mechanism than do pharmaceutical drugs, thus it can help in situations where conventional drugs have not worked.[4]

The question remains, however, as to how cannabis does reduce this pressure. The dam analogy may again aid our understanding. The floodgates are shut, the river is blocked, and it overflows its banks. Similarly, blocked eye ducts lead to a backup of ocular fluids. As an engineer would open up the floodgates to release water and lower the water level, so orthodox medicine seeks to reopen these ducts and drain the excess fluid. Nature's gentler alternative is to let the water spread out and be absorbed into marshes that suck the water down into an underground water table. Similarly, instead of opening the valves, cannabis dehydrates the eyes, thereby reducing the volume of fluid that is trying to pass through them. This reduces the pressure, saving the eye and maintaining healthy vision for years on end.

Cannabis is at least as effective in reducing eye pressure as are currently legal medicines, but without toxic side effects, change in eye color, or damage to the liver and kidneys, all of which have been associated with presently approved glaucoma drugs. Cannabis can be smoked or eaten to reduce the pressure. Both clinical studies and practical experience bear this out. When faced with a patient whose vision and ocular structure have been destroyed by glaucoma, few would withhold whatever relief an herb can provide.

VIEWING THE WORLD
THROUGH ROSE-COLORED EYES

Robert S. Hepler, M.D., first prescribed marijuana in 1975 for Robert Randall, a glaucoma patient facing imminent blindness. Randall had long been aware that just before his eye pressure went out of control, he saw rainbow outlines around lights. He inadvertently discovered that if he smoked cannabis, those auras disappeared—and his eye pressure dropped. Randall subjectively recognized that there was a connection between those two occurrences. Unfortunately, the police discovered his house plants, took his medicine away, and arrested him. Randall had to prove in court that his use of marijuana was a matter of medical necessity.

The option of surgery carried with it unacceptable risks. Available drugs were inadequate to control his eye pressure. Dr. Hepler measured the patient's IOP levels, and found that large doses of smoked marijuana effectively reduced Randall's pressure into a safe range over the course of an entire test day. He concluded that the only known alternative to preserve the patient's remaining eyesight would be to include cannabis as part of this regular medical regimen. The judge agreed, and Randall became the first person to receive medical marijuana from the government as part of the federal Compassionate Investigational New Drug (IND) program. John Merritt, M.D., and Richard North, M.D., treated Randall and monitored his condition over the years. More than a decade later, they testified to DEA administrative law judge Francis Young that they were convinced that the patient's ongoing use of cannabis had saved his fragile eyesight. Robert Randall's case history helped the judge determine in 1988 that cannabis is a safe and effective medicine for the treatment of glaucoma.[5] In 1996, more than twenty years after being told that he was about to go blind, Randall still smokes cannabis every day, and he still can see.

Elvy Musikka had congenital cataracts and other eye problems from early childhood. As her already bad eyesight continued to deteriorate, she endured prescription pharmaceutical drugs that had uncomfortable side effects but little benefit, and eye surgeries that resulted in glaucoma by early adulthood. She tried drug after drug, experiencing a "nightmare" of side effects. Turning to ever more desperate measures, she underwent a risky surgery on her better, right eye. The operation left her blinded in that eye.

Desperate to save the little sight she had in her other failing eye, she finally stopped resisting suggestions that she use marijuana to reduce her IOP. To her grudging surprise, she found that it seemed to work. Musikka discussed the situation with her doctor, conducting her own experiments by eating marijuana brownies before certain visits to the doctor. His measurements verified that the herb did, indeed, bring down her eye pressure.

Elvy decided to grow her own plants so as to remove herself from the underground market, and found that she had a green thumb. That was enough to attract the attention of the police, who arrested her. Elvy argued medical necessity and the judge agreed to hear the testimony. That's when she learned that her doctors had never made notes on her observations about cannabis. She had to rely on the testimony of expert witnesses and her new physician, who testified that smoking marijuana did make a measurable difference in her eye pressure, and that nothing else had been effective. The judge ruled in her favor, stating that Elvy "would have to be insane" to forego the use of medical marijuana. She was placed on the federal IND program.

Musikka continues to receive three hundred government-prepared marijuana cigarettes to smoke each month, more than one for every two waking hours. Even though they are not as good as the medicine she once grew herself, Elvy Musikka maintains that her vision has actually improved, thanks to her steady use of cannabis for twenty years. She is an avid crusader for medical rights who expresses her outrage that other patients are denied access to a medicine that has helped her so much. "I didn't lose my eyesight to glaucoma," says Elvy. "I lost it to ignorance."

OTHER EFFECTS OF
CANNABIS ON THE EYES

Bloodshot eyes are a highly consistent physical indication of resination.[6] This phenomenon appears with smoked doses as low as 2.5 mg THC.[7] Using an 18-mg dose, Dr. Andrew Weil found such reddening in all frequent cannabis users and in eight out of nine inexperienced subjects.[8] People with conjunctivitis, or inflamed eyes, might take this into consideration before smoking cannabis, but as yet there is no data to suggest any real risk. The reddening of the eyes is not caused by ruptures in blood vessels, but by dilation of the vessels, which makes them more visible. There are eye drops available that constrict these capillaries again, to hide the redness, but their use is not recommended.

Researchers have found neither impairment nor improvement in objective visual acuity or in the perception of light brightness, testing both naive and experienced users at smoked doses of four to six mg THC.[9] Other studies demonstrated that there was no effect on depth perception, duration of after-image, or visual motor coordination tests. Conventional wisdom once held that cannabis dilated the pupils and some early studies had reported enlarged pupils and a sluggish reaction to light.[10] However, when pupil diameter was systematically measured, researchers found no dilation at doses up to 70 mg. To the contrary, sophisticated instrumentation has demonstrated a slight but consistent pupillary constriction within five minutes of smoking.[11] A preservation of normal light responsiveness is common, followed in a few hours by a depression of pupillary responsiveness to nearby stimulation, possibly representing fatigue or sleepiness. One study identified a consistent increase in glare recovery time, which persisted for several hours but was not dose related.[12] Further tests revealed that this was not related to change in illumination threshold or pupil size.

This extra sensitivity to light, which manifests itself in dark settings, may explain the mechanism behind another possible benefit attributed to cannabis use: improved night vision. M. E. West of the University of the West Indies in Kingston, Jamaica, observed that local fishermen who smoke cannabis or drink an alcoholic beverage made with the stems and leaves of the plant have "an uncanny ability to see in the dark."[13] However, factors such as practice and familiarity with the situation cannot be fully discounted in this observation.

The only eye anomaly that has been established as a pattern among long-term, heavy cannabis users is a slight yellow discoloration of the eye caused by permanent congestion of the transverse ciliary vessels, as observed in the cannabis culture of India.[14] This probably has to do with the ongoing dehydration of the eye. The use of lubricating eye drops may help to mitigate this effect. A few patients have experienced rare and peculiar responses, not all of which are desirable. There are anecdotal reports of swollen eyelids, drooping upper eyelids, hyper-sensitivity to light, and rapid, involuntary eye movements.[15] Such responses are quite rare, and stop when their consumption of cannabis is discontinued.

A recommended remedy for headaches due to tired or weak eyes combines cannabis tincture with that of nucis vomicus taken several times per day.[16] Cannabis also acts as a nervous sedative in exophthalmic goiter. This is a protrusion of one or both eyeballs exposing an unusually large amount of the front of the eye, resulting in a staring appearance. It is usually caused by thyrotoxicosis, an over-active and swollen thyroid gland that is often a result of iodine deficiency, disease, or the side-effect of some drug. This is an example of how an effect experienced as a negative by one user—droopy eyelids—may compensate for a condition and be perceived as a benefit by another patient.

It all depends on how you look at it.

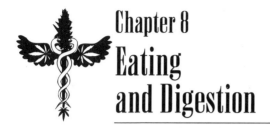# Chapter 8
Eating
and Digestion

Hemp crosses paths with the human gastronomic system in four ways. First, its seed is used as a primary food source, and the seed oil can be pressed out to be added to food as a dietary supplement. Second, it is possible to eat the resinous foliage of marijuana and take advantage of its medicinal benefits without smoking. Third, smoked cannabis helps soothe the stomach and prevents vomiting. And fourth, cannabis may change the very nature of the relationship an individual patient has with food.

This last effect is one of the most important benefits of medical marijuana, yet one that is rarely taken seriously. It's called "the munchies" in the vernacular. That term covers a wide range of effects that have led to countless jokes about marijuana smokers. You take a few puffs. Your mouth begins to dry out a bit, making you want to consume something to moisten your palate. Next comes almost a craving for food, or at least an insatiable curiosity as to what might be available to eat, if you *did* feel like eating something. After that comes the experimental appetite, in which something you ordinarily would not eat suddenly becomes very appealing . . . or at least worth giving another chance. And once the eating begins, you find a new world of tastes and flavors that triggers a fantastic appreciation of food and unleashes a voracious desire to consume more and more, until someone finally has to pry the peanut butter jar out of your hands at two in the morning.

To many people, however, being able to hold down food and get proper nutrition is no joking matter. When there is no appetite or desire to eat, there is less intake of raw materials for the body to rebuild damaged systems. When a patient can't hold food down, they can't eat properly. And if you don't eat, you die. It's that simple. Resinous cannabis stimulates the appetite and helps patients with debilitating conditions eat and thereby gain weight, giving them the strength they need to combat disease or infection, and to effect a recovery. Cannabis and its extracts have demonstrated clinical utility in treating persons with *anorexia nervosa*, as well as the wasting syndrome associated with tuberculosis, AIDS, and cancer. The herb has also proven useful in settling the stomachs of people with problems such as motion sickness. Its euphoric effect also raises a patient's spirits, improving overall chances of survival and recovery.

This use of cannabis is well established in the classical literature and in folk remedy, although controlled studies of the effect are still lacking due to bureaucratic interference in doing the necessary research. The following patient's case history goes back to the days before marijuana prohibition began. "As a child about six years old I had developed a severe nausea from some form of germ or virus. My mother took me to see a Finnish doctor in New York. He prepared some herbs in a container, lit them, and with a towel draped over my head I was told to breathe in the smoke. As I remember, it cleared up the nausea and I recovered soon thereafter. This took place about 1933, and I understood it to be an old practice in Finland. It wasn't until one day I surprised my kids smoking 'pot' that I recognized that smell. There should be references to that medical use in Finland and other European countries."

Of course, such traditional references do exist,[1] but many of the health problems for which cannabis has proven most effective are relatively new, such as cancer and AIDS.

COPING WITH LIFE DURING CANCER

Cancer is an environmentally-caused disease in which the body's natural defense systems are overridden and possibly turned against the patient. Normal cells have growth restraints; cancer cells do not. The resulting development of uncontrolled tissue growths, called tumors, can become malignant and spread through various body systems. These invaders grow at a rapid and painful rate, squeezing out healthy tissues, causing intense pain, and interfering with normal functioning of the body. In most cases, cancer is an age-related phenomenon, so personal risk increases with the individual's age. Over the coming years, cancer will strike an estimated one out of five Americans and affect three out of four families. About a hundred million Americans now living will develop cancer, and in many cases this will prove terminal. There is, as yet, no cure for cancer. That is why it is important to put the disease into remission in a way that allows a high degree of comfort and normalcy. Cannabis helps make living with cancer easier and more dignified.

My father, Robert Conrad, was one of the unlucky ones. He died of cancer on Christmas Eve of 1994. During his final illness, he was kept at a Veterans Administration hospital in upstate New York, where the doctors gave him a variety of opiates and other pharmaceuticals. These hard drugs were able to control most of his pain, but he suffered a variety of side effects including constipation, lack of appetite, upset stomach, irritability, restlessness, insomnia, confusion, and what he called a "mental fog" that made his conversations disjointed and occasionally incoherent. A fiercely independent man, he was distressed to find himself confined to a wheelchair and hospital bed. We discussed some of the data that showed cannabis could help relieve most of his symptoms. He was interested. "I'll gladly be the guinea pig to test the stuff out," he remarked. "What have I got to lose?" His physician, however, refused even to seriously discuss the use of cannabis as an adjunct to treatment. When my father found out I had mentioned it to his doctor, he became afraid to use the herb, lest it be reported to the police. He continued to deteriorate. I visited him at a picnic table under a large tree growing on the hospital grounds, discussing life and memories. When he was in exceptional misery, I again suggested cannabis. He refused, and warned me not to take any more risks for him. I still remember one of the last conversations I had with him, when he took me by the arm and looked into my eyes with intense inner pain and desperation. "It's just not right," he told me. "No one should have to go through this. Promise me something, Chris. Promise you'll do something to legalize medical marijuana, and make sure no one else has to suffer like this." When I agreed, he squeezed my arm and nodded his approval. I returned to California. Soon after that he took a turn for the worse, and did not recover. I never saw my dad alive again after that day.

Among the worst experiences many cancer patients cite are the terrible side effects of the most common nonsurgical treatments—radiation and chemotherapy. The problem is that these powerful therapies not only damage cancer tissues but affect healthy tissues as well, leaving the patient in a painful and debilitated state. The treatments often cause reactions that lead to uncontrollable vomiting, which forces all the food out of a patient's belly and may still continue for hours afterward with convulsive "dry heaves" that leave the patient crumpled on the floor in pain. As the duration of the treatment becomes longer, the cumulative effect can be devastating. While using powerful pain killers, the patient will often lose the ability to eat or rest properly, which can bring on another group of health and psychological problems, or even make the difference between life and death. Some patients discontinue the treatment because they cannot stand its physical toll.

Cannabis boosts patients' spirits, helps them to eat and combat the excessive weight loss of wasting syndrome, and is also a potent antiemetic. Just a few puffs of a marijuana cigarette can drastically reduce or even completely eliminate the gut-wrenching nausea triggered by chemotherapy and radiation treatments.[2] Some of this benefit may stem from the resin's antispasmodic effect, which suppresses the gag reflex and relaxes abdominal muscle spasms. Whatever the mechanism it follows, studies on cancer patients who smoked cannabis under medical supervision in New Mexico, California, Michigan, New York, Georgia, and Tennessee found that cannabis often reduced nausea and vomiting when all available prescription drugs failed to work.[3] A majority of cancer specialists from around the country who responded to a 1991 Harvard University survey agreed that doctors should be allowed to prescribe natural cannabis for their patients.[4] Smoking is an extremely effective delivery system, preferred by patients and doctors alike.[5] A survey of cancer patients undergoing chemotherapy found that most of them said that smoked marijuana was much more effective in controlling nausea than synthetic THC pills. Smoked cannabis is also less expensive and more practical since, unlike a pill, it cannot be vomited up. It is also less likely than THC to cause unpleasant side effects, because the compounds in natural cannabis that act as buffers, such as cannabidiol, are not included in the pill.

James Cox was first introduced to marijuana following two operations for testicular cancer that had metastasized to his stomach. He found that smoking it helped him cope with the pain, nausea, and eating disorders resulting from not only his cancer, but also his chemotherapy and radiation treatments, and it helped restore his appetite. He was also prescribed Demerol, which, in combination with cannabis, relieved the chronic pain due to nerve damage in his stomach and other organs. James was on the pharmaceutical for fifteen years and became addicted. By increasing his cannabis intake he was able to get off the Demerol and regain control of his life. Police twice found his Missouri marijuana garden, confiscated his medicine, and, the second time, the courts locked him away. Deprived of cannabis, James's health problems returned with a vengeance. He found himself unable to eat, and his health quickly deteriorated. His weight plunged to dangerous levels. "Since I have been incarcerated and deprived of its use I have lived in constant discomfort and I feel this is a direct result of not having the medical benefits of marijuana. My stomach deteriorated to the point to where I could not eat anything due to incurable bleeding ulcers," James wrote. It took two major stomach surgeries for James to be able to put on weight again and return to the level he had maintained through his previous regular use of cannabis.[6] He is still denied access to medical marijuana.

Cannabis extracts have been directly applied to tumors to shrink their size and possibly stop them from spreading.[7] However, currently cannabis is only being used as an adjunct to the conventional treatments that are offered.

AIDS AND HIV DISORDERS

The same healing characteristics that benefit cancer patients are also utilized by thousands of patients with Acquired Immunodeficiency Syndrome (AIDS) or Human Immunodeficiency Virus (HIV). The body responds to the HIV invasion just as it responds to a burn, tumor, or surgery. It demands extra nourishment, and, if necessary, it begins to break down the protein stored in the body's own muscles. Patients are instructed to eat enough to avoid weight loss, which occurs in 98 percent of HIV cases. To compensate they should get almost twice as much protein intake as a healthy individual.[8]

Many people with AIDS report improved appetite and weight gain after they begin smoking cannabis. Kenneth Jenks was a hemophiliac living in Florida who contracted AIDS through a blood transfusion and then passed it on to his wife, Barbara, before he was aware of what had happened. Both were suffering from nausea, vomiting, and appetite loss caused by AIDS or the AZT therapy. The doctor feared that Barbara would die of starvation. In early 1989 the couple learned about marijuana through a support group for people with AIDS. Desperate for anything that would help, they began to smoke cannabis. They felt better, regained some weight, and were able to stay out of the hospital for about a year before an anonymous informant sent the police to their door on March 29, 1990. The police found the two small plants the couple had been growing in order to save money. The Jenks argued medical necessity in court, and the defense was rejected, but the appeals court overturned the decision and sustained the medical necessity defense. They were placed into the Investigational New Drug (IND) program and given free government-grown marijuana. The publicity around their case led to hundreds of AIDS patients petitioning the Food and Drug Administration to be let into the program. Because of this attention, the program was terminated on June 21, 1991. Government officials have since maintained that it would be inappropriate to make a medical exception for AIDS patients to use cannabis, because they fear the risk of *aspergillus* mold growing on the herb and causing lung infections. Moldy cannabis should not be smoked by anyone. Any suspect cannabis should be heated in an oven for at least three minutes at 220°F. Although that will overdry the herb, it will kill any bacteria.

People with AIDS who use cannabis regularly report that the drug allows them to continue to live a more normal life with relatively few side effects. Powerful testimonials and case histories are being documented at AIDS clinics and cannabis buyers clubs across the country.

So, how does it work? Reports of increased hunger, especially for sweets, during cannabis resination have focused attention on possible changes in blood sugar level, often with contradictory results.[9] Early investigators reported decreases, but later studies found slight increases, no change at all, and movement in both directions.[10] L. E. Hollister found that reports of appetite stimulation and subjective hunger occurred in slightly more than half of his subjects.[11] He found a significant increase in total food intake after 26 mg of THC were ingested when the subject had eaten breakfast—but not when the subject was fasting. It's a mixed bag. While most people seem to increase their appetite by smoking cannabis, I have talked to a significant number who smoke as a way of suppressing their appetites. Once again, personal experience is the best way to determine how cannabis works for you.

Despite all the research that has been done—or perhaps because of all the research that has been prevented[12]—we still know very little about the how and why of cannabis's amazing calming-yet-stimulating effect on the human digestive system. Is it physiological or is it neurological? More research is desperately needed, but we don't need to understand *why* cannabis works to know that it *does* work. The important thing is that these patients regain access to this resinous herb and determine with their physicians, rather than adminstrators in Washington, D.C., whether cannabis is the right medicine for them. Now *there's* food for thought.

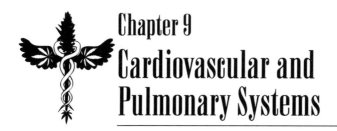

Chapter 9
Cardiovascular and Pulmonary Systems

Smoking is by far the most popular method of consuming resinous cannabis. Many people simply enjoy the flavor. They might smoke the flower as an appetizer before dinner, or use it to cleanse the palate before dessert. The smoking process is also a remarkably fast and efficient delivery system. The particles of smoke that carry the active resinous compounds are so small that they are inhaled with the breath to the depths of the lung, where the drug is instantly absorbed across the alveolar membrane into the bloodstream.

By directly introducing cannabis drugs into the heart–lung *(cardio-pulmonary)* interchange, you get them into the bloodstream, up through the aorta, and into the brain without being diluted or passing through the liver. Blood flows into the heart by way of the *vena cava.* The ventricle chamber on the right side of the heart pumps "used" blood through the pulmonary artery to the lungs, where the alveoli transfer the carbon dioxide to be exhaled, and replace it with oxygen and whatever else has been taken into the lungs. The reoxygenated blood flows back through the pulmonary veins to the left atrium, through the mitral valve and into the left ventricle chamber, which contracts and pushes the blood out through the aorta to the brain and the rest of the body. To illustrate the virtue of smoking as a delivery system, in one trial 10–15 mg of smoked THC measured a peak concentration about eight times as great as that which followed 20 mg eaten THC, and in much less time.[1]

The heart and circulatory system combined make up the cardiovascular system; the core of inner vitality and the flow of life. Fresh blood leaves the heart in a surge, and returns to it through miles of vessels that range in size from large arteries to minute capillaries. Blood continuously flows out into the body through the arteries and then returns back to the heart through the veins. Along this route, blood cells feed oxygen, nutrients, and medicinal compounds to the body's other cells as they pick up waste materials that will be disposed through the liver into urine or fecal matter. Pressure to drive the hard-working blood on its commute through the vascular system comes from rhythmic cardiac contractions—the steady pumping of the heart. This life-giving cadence causes the pulse to beat at a measurable rate.

One of the most consistent physical effects of consuming resinous cannabis, whether it is smoked or eaten, is an increase in the pulse rate. This change is sufficiently dose-related and reproducible with both the natural herb and pure THC to stand as an objective measurement of cannabis's overall effect.[2] Reported increases have ranged from 10 to 40 beats per minute in response to THC doses ranging from 2 to 70 mg.[3] After using this herb a few times, the patient becomes familiar with the stimulant effect and soon learns to accept or even look forward to it. The pulse effect diminishes in regular herb smokers over the course of a few weeks, showing that a low level of tolerance has developed. It continues to occur, however, regardless of the patient's experience with marijuana. Oral doses of clonidine, taken three hours before consuming cannabis, suppressed this cardiovascular response without reducing the herb's psychoactive effects.[4] However, the massive doses of resin consumed for religious purposes in India were reported to significantly slow the heartbeats of ascetics.[5] Extreme doses of cannabis tincture were found to slow the breath rate considerably, and enormous amounts have been given to animals without causing a lethal effect.[6]

Consuming cannabis stimulates cardiovascular activity by speeding up the heart rate while expanding the blood vessels. It acts as a vasodilator, meaning the compounds in the resin open up the blood vessels.[7] This facilitates blood flow throughout the vascular system, which may lower the blood pressure and help reduce stress. The patient's overall body temperature remains essentially unchanged or may be slightly lowered, and a noticeable cooling of the digits and extremities is not uncommon. This is probably why cannabis is so often recommended to lower a patient's fever in classical medical literature. Certain THC analogs may also prove quite valuable for treating high blood pressure and uncontrollable fevers.[8] Such benefits are temporary, lasting only as long as the active compounds are in the blood stream, but would often be sufficient to get the patient safely through a crisis situation.

STRESS REDUCTION

Many social users say that they use marijuana to unwind, and quite a few have confided that there have been situations when smoking some cannabis kept them from blowing their stack. Cannabis aids psychological perspective, which helps to make the little nuisances of life just that much less irritating. The importance of this function is often underrated, for high stress can kill. A high tension lifestyle carries its own price tag in terms of heart disease and social interaction. Hostile people are about twice as likely to suffer from heart disease and to die from any cause. "People who are hostile are at risk of getting divorced, more likely to be alone, less likely to take care of their health, and more likely to be heavy drinkers," said Todd Q. Miller, assistant professor of preventive medicine at the University of Texas Medical Branch at Galveston, Texas. He suggested that

"reprogramming" one's outlook could be as effective a prevention tool as exercising, avoiding cigarettes, and eating right. The
findings come from a statistical analysis of forty-five reports link-
ing heart disease and death to hostility. Now, it appears, their
psychological profile also makes them more likely to become ill
and die. Cannabis offers such high-strung personalities a relatively safe way to unwind before their situation hits a crisis point.
Furthermore, the pattern of deep breathing plus breath control that is associated with smoking cannabis may serve as a form
of relaxation therapy that reduces stress and generates a sub-
lime sense of well-being.

Apparently THC produces little or no electrocardiographic
abnormalities or changes in circulation rate. Reports on the effects of a wide range of dosages on blood pressure are inconsis-
tent. Some investigators using pure THC have reported slight
decreases in blood pressure, while others reported minor increases. Still others have been unable to demonstrate any significant effect, using smoked or oral preparations. L. E. Hollister
analyzed blood and urine samples subsequent to oral administration of either THC or synhexyl.[9] Total white blood cell count
increased and overall redness of the fluid decreased, but no significant changes were found in platelet serotonin content, plasma
cortisol level, or urinary catecholamine excretion. These findings indicate that cannabis has no major effect on these common physical measures of stress. Other studies looked at possible blood chemistry changes, using from 7.5 mg to 75 mg THC
equivalent.[10] They found no changes in total white blood cell
count, red blood cell structure or number, or the ratio between
the two. Furthermore, no significant change was detected in
platelet count; reticulocyte count; blood urea nitrogen; concentration of sodium, potassium, chloride, bicarbonate, calcium,
or phosphorous; liver function tests; protein electrophoresis; or
uric acid concentration.

The accelerated heartbeat has been mentioned as a possible
contraindication against the use of cannabis drugs by people

with heart conditions, although there is no empirical data to support that concern. From a practical viewpoint, the most common negative effect is when people who are unfamiliar with this effect become aware of their speeded up heartbeat and start to worry about it. Their concern causes emotional tension, which increases the heartbeat again. That response compounds their fear and anxiety, which increases the heartbeat yet again and that pattern could ultimately trigger a brief, but unpleasant, panic attack. This does not pose any physical danger to a healthy individual. Many people have briefly experienced this without any harmful consequences, and there is no cause for serious concern. The best remedy is to calm down. Sit back, breathe deeply, relax, and talk to someone you feel comfortable with or do something to take your mind off your heartbeat while you wait for the anxiety to pass.

Remember, a vigorous heartbeat is a good sign. It means you're alive.

AIR PASSAGES AND ASTHMA

Cannabis smoke is an excellent dilator of the tiny air tubes in the lungs called the bronchi and the bronchioles, opening them up to allow more oxygen into the blood.[11] These air passages attach to the alveoli, the roughly 400 million tiny air sacs in the lungs where the oxygen exchange takes place. The amount of oxygen the blood can carry is at its maximum at around age fifty. After that, the lungs gradually lose elasticity and the alveoli thicken, impeding the passage of gases across the membranes. Ultimately, more air has to be breathed to properly oxygenate the blood, and overall breathing capacity is diminished by up to 40 percent by age seventy.[12] Research into the lungs' oxygen transfer mechanism suggests that, since cannabis smoke is a bronchodilator, the shallowness of breath, headaches, chest pains, and other symptoms of exposure to heavy smog might be somewhat alleviated by moderate use of cannabis. It is conceivable that regular cannabis smoking could slow the aging process of the lungs themselves.

Asthma is a pulmonary condition characterized by attacks of breathlessness and wheezing, caused by constriction of the bronchioles. About ten million Americans have asthma, and it kills more than four thousand in a typical year. The five thousand deaths attributed to it in 1995 represent a 44 percent increase since 1983. It starts when a simple inhalation picks up any of a number of irritants, such as pollen, dust, feathers, or animal hair and dander. This sets off allergic reactions, which are aggravated by cold air, infections, exercise, and air pollution. The muscles surrounding the bronchial tubes contract and squeeze the flow of air. The linings of the bronchioles swell and become inflamed. The air passages become even narrower. They fill with phlegm, and muscle spasms trigger coughing fits. Eventually a chronic cough may develop. In severe cases, a combination of steroids and bronchodilators may be prescribed.

Contrary to what one might expect, smoking cannabis can actually relieve asthma by relaxing the bronchial muscles and expanding the bronchioles. This facilitates the exchange of gases within the lungs and increases the total oxygen flow. The smoke acts very quickly, and a few puffs can bring fast relief to an asthmatic attack. A study by Dr. Donald Tashkin showed that both natural cannabis and THC improved the flow of air into the lungs, and that while certain pharmaceutical bronchodilators worked faster with a stronger peak effect, the effect of THC lasted longer and had fewer side effects.[13]

Joe Pinson is a lifelong asthma patient. His mother, Regina, and his grandmother, Amy Paterson, can testify to the time they spent taking care of Joe as a child. They recount the many times they had to rush him to the hospital as he was turning gray, because he could not breathe due to his severe, life-threatening bouts with asthma. He missed so much school one year that he was held back a grade, and his family got him a private tutor to work at home. Drug after pharmaceutical drug failed to help much. Then, at age eighteen, his episodes suddenly and mysteriously stopped. For the first time, he could breathe and lead a normal life. His family was so relieved that he had finally grown out of his asthma. What his family didn't know was that Joe had discovered that smoking resinous cannabis could stop an asthma attack in its tracks. He could go from gasping for breath to relatively normal breathing with just a few puffs of the pungent smoke. He kept this a secret, and decided that the best way to keep anyone from finding out would be to stop buying cannabis on the street. Federal agents began to investigate Joe in 1991 after he bought some indoor gardening equipment, and they later found marijuana plants in his attic. He was given a five-year mandatory minimum sentence for growing his own medicine. In prison, Joe is deprived of the natural medicine that has proven the most effective for controlling his asthma. Instead, he is given hard drugs, such as steroids, with known harmful side effects.[14]

LUNG IRRITATION AND BRONCHITIS

Cannabis smoke contains components that cause small, temporary lesions in the lining of the lungs, which heal quickly with no demonstrated long-term effect. There is no evidence that such damage has ever led to lung cancer; however, common sense dictates caution, and heavy smoking has been repeatedly shown to increase the likelihood of contracting bronchitis. This risk is greater in areas with more polluted air. If this happens to you, the treatment is simple: Stop smoking, and the problem will go away. What superficial damage cannabis smoke does to the human lung is limited to the large air passage, not the more fragile bronchi and alveoli. If a patient has bronchitis, emphysema, or any other lung problem, however, it is probably not a good idea to smoke anything—not even cannabis. In an attempt to eliminate this problem, THC was isolated and administered to asthma patients in an aerosol form to relax bronchospasms. Unfortunately the aerosols themselves proved to be irritating, and fell

Comparison of Cannabis Delivery Systems

Method of application	Advantages	Disadvantages
Creams, lotions, salves	Condition skin or soothes inflammation	Limited to superficial and external applications
Dronabinol (Marinol)	Legally prescribable THC	Expensive, synthetic, lacks other synergistic cannabinoids
Eaten herb in food, pills, capsules	Long lasting effect; subtly different than smoked cannabis; easily prepared; no pulmonary irritation	Must be heated; difficult to gauge dosage
Eaten hempseed	Nutritional and immune support; gentle to system	Long-term consumption required to get full benefits; sterilization of seed in U.S. slightly reduces nutritive benefits
Smoked herb or derivative	Almost immediate effect; easy to gauge effects and titrate dosage; easily prepared and consumed	Irritates pulmonary system
Suppositories	Rapid assimilation of medicine without smoking or eating	Very anal; not yet available on the market
Tinctures	Easy oral preparation	Contains alcohol; not available in standard dosages; difficult to judge quality
Vaporizer	Same rapid onset of effects typical of smoked medicine, but without the extra health hazards of smoke	Requires special equipment

into disuse. A new inhalation device, known as a vaporizer, heats the cannabis to the point where its essence is released in a vapor before the plant matter begins to burn. This offers exciting new possibilities in treatment.

When cannabis is legal prices will drop significantly, and people will be able to afford more potent strains, to take shorter inhalations, and to use vaporizers, water pipes, and other systems that minimize possible damage. In the meantime, for safer consumption, the patient should try not to inhale so deeply when smoking, and should take in more fresh air and exhale sooner. Due to the efficiency of the THC transfer through smoking, most medical benefits are received almost instantly, and any loss of effects from not holding the smoke in will be minimal compared to the reduced health risk.

While much ado has been made of the possible risks of the smoking process, the amount of research on this aspect of cannabis use is skewed and misleading; it has been exaggerated in an effort to rationalize drug policies against cannabis. And don't forget that in most cases cannabis need not be smoked at all. Although smoking cannabis is a much faster and more efficient way of getting relief, most of the benefits can be enjoyed by eating it as well. If it is eaten, there is no negative effect on the respiratory tissues.

OTHER CHARACTERISTICS OF CANNABIS SMOKE

Jamaican and Costa Rican studies looked at very heavy, regular cannabis smokers and found no significant difference in respiratory health to distinguish them from the non-smoking control group. Researchers using electron microscopic methods were able to detect damage in the pulmonary tree of tobacco smokers, but found no such damage among short- or even long-term cannabis smokers.[15]

On the other hand, cannabis smoke is an expectorant that helps the patient break up and expel phlegm and clear out congested air passages. Cannabis resin is also helpful in suppressing coughs. It was reported in the 1920s that cannabis tincture is "one of the best additions to cough mixtures that we possess, as it quiets that tickling in the throat, and yet does not constipate nor depress the system as does morphine."[16]

Dryness of the mouth and throat are typical symptoms of cannabis consumption. Oral dehydration occurs whether the cannabis is smoked or eaten, but the effect is most pronounced when smoked. The use of throat lozenges or chewing gum moistens the patient's palate, but shortly afterwards the dryness returns. Drinking water has relatively little effect in reducing this dryness. It is possible that the oily smoke may coat the surface of the mouth with a sticky, resinous film that temporarily prevents saliva from replenishing the surface moisture in the mouth. On the other hand, the herb's diuretic action may actually be siphoning off the saliva to flush out the body. Apart from being a minor inconvenience, the only notable negative effects of oral dehydration, commonly known as "cotton mouth," are dry kisses and the need to take a drink before speaking.

There are several therapeutic applications of this phenomenon. One is to dry the mouth in order to facilitate a particular medical process, such as visiting the dentist—a situation in which cannabis's analgesic and relaxing properties may also help. Cotton mouth also encourages one to drink more liquids, thereby flushing out one's entire system. Another use is to dry out the mucus linings of the nasal cavity when one has a runny nose. This is achieved by inhaling the smoke up through the nose to dehydrate the mucus membranes, and it may also have a local anti-inflammatory effect.

Your body is a temple. Don't be afraid to burn a little incense.

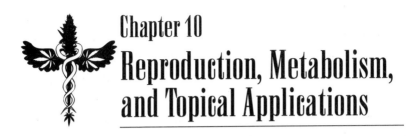

Chapter 10
Reproduction, Metabolism, and Topical Applications

REPRODUCTION AND CHILDBIRTH

An early warning about cannabis and childbirth comes from a European explorer's note that some Ugandan superstitions forbade married women to smoke cannabis because of the effect it could have upon either her or her child, "should she be about to become a mother."[1] Modern studies have found little to worry about in this regard—concentrations of inert THC cannabinoids in the testes and ovaries of cannabis smokers are among the lowest measured in any body organs.[2] Nonetheless, most orthodox physicians discourage pregnant women from smoking cannabis. Cannabinoids cross the placenta, and conventional wisdom dictates that a pregnant woman take extraordinary care not to expose her unborn child to any perceived risks.

Traditionally, however, cannabis flowers were an important part of the midwife's basket of remedies, used to ease labor. Cannabis has long been used to control the nausea of morning sickness. A fourth-century tomb near Jerusalem yielded physical evidence that cannabis was used in the birthing process. Israeli archaeologists stumbled upon a 1600-year-old tragedy—the remains of a narrow-hipped, teenage woman still bearing the skeleton of a full-term fetus in her abdomen. In the chamber with her was a dish of gray ashes that contained charred cannabis seeds and traces of THC.[3] Could it be that her midwife had administered the plant in a desperate effort to bring on labor and ease the pain? If so, it would not have been unusual. The plant's resin was valued in ancient Persia for treating miscarriages. The Sotho women of Africa traditionally smoke the herb during childbirth to speed up their labor, and their children are fed ground-up seed with bread or mealy-pap for weaning.[4] The Chinese *Pen T'sao Kang Mu* also prescribed the use of hempseed for such things as an aid in sterility and miscarriage. It cited a passage from the older work, *Ri Hua* or *The Essence of Daily Life*, that called for hempseed remedies in the following circumstances. "It will bring benefit in every and all types of malignancy. . . . It will increase the flow of mother's milk for the suckling of infants. It has the capacity to quench thirst. It can be used to hasten childbirth, where the delivery is troubled with complications, or overdue."[5]

Use of resinous cannabis extracts continued to be important throughout the nineteenth century in treating women and mothers-to-be. The *United States Dispensatory* of 1854 noted its value for treating uterine hemorrhage. It added that it had the properties of "hastening and increasing the contractions of the uterus in delivery. . . . [I]t acts very quickly, and without anesthetic effect."[6] Cannabis extract was also described in the *British Medical Journal* for controlling menorrhagia (excessive menstrual bleeding) as "a valuable aid to diagnosis in cases in which it is uncertain whether an early abortion may or may not have occurred."[7] Its common use in the past encouraged an anonymous modern-day couple to have a hemp childbirth, including plenty of hempseed essential fatty acids in the diet and hempseed oil massages to lubricate the vaginal opening and keep the skin moisturized as it stretched for the birth. The mother ate some cannabis to relax her uterine muscles and in the last moments smoked to ease the pain of the contractions. The couple was very satisfied with the results of their home birthing experiment, and the child is healthy, bright, happy, and growing up well.

The resin of cannabis has been recommended as a diversion for those prone to alcohol abuse, to stimulate conversation, and to excite sensuality between marriage partners. Frederick Hollick's *Marriage Guide* recommended the consumption of hashish for marriages in trouble, since it was a sexual stimulant "of extraordinary power."[8] In sexual impotence not caused by disease, cannabis was prescribed in combination with strychnine or nux vomica and ergot. It appears that cannabis's reputation as a sexual stimulant, described in great detail in the ancient Hindu *Bhagavat-purana,*[9] has both physical and psychological aspects.[10] Measurements of the testes of dogs who were given cannabis resin found that the resulting vascular dilatation increased blood supply to the gonads, which researchers associated with increased glandular activity and concluded that, "it is probable that, in this sense, hemp should be regarded as a true aphrodisiac."[11] However, it was further noted that the dogs did not behave as if they were under the influence of an aphrodisiac. Hence, the mechanism in cannabis that causes sexual arousal in humans might be psychological rather than physical. Once the initial arousal is achieved, the vasodilation will continue to enhance the flow of blood to the genitalia, thereby filling out the erection in the male and stimulating the production of vaginal fluids in the female. Cannabis does not, however, lead to the uncontrollable sexual urges implied by the old "reefer madness" anti-marijuana propaganda. Individuals remain in full control of, and fully responsible for, their activities.

METABOLISM, ELIMINATION, AND DISPOSAL

What goes in must come out, and cannabis is no exception to the rule. The body acts quickly to reject and expel harmful foreign substances, if necessary by vomiting or diarrhea. Benign substances, on the other hand, are processed slowly, so the body can utilize any possible nutritional or medicinal compounds.

Cannabis is so safe and nontoxic that the body is in no hurry to get rid of it. Human metabolism regards cannabinoids like butter or any other fatty compound that has been consumed by the patient. It has even been suggested that this slow disposal process explains why it is virtually impossible to become physically addicted to cannabis; the cannabinoids don't leave the system fast enough to cause severe withdrawal symptoms such as painful cravings.[12] Both eaten and smoked cannabis are detectable for days in the feces and for weeks in the urine, long after resination wears off.[13] It leaves a long-term trace in human hair that can be detected for years on end.

Immediately after being inhaled as smoke, cannabinoids are transferred to the blood, carried to the left heart chamber, and shipped out to the arteries. From here the THC is mixed with a relatively small volume of arterial blood and pumped directly to the brain. Cerebral blood flow is large, and the brain is a fatty organ, so THC is promptly absorbed into the lipids of the brain tissue, which initiates the psychoactive experience. The rapid buildup of active compounds in the brain is followed by their steady reduction. This process explains the relative intensity and brevity of the peak effect, which is followed by an extended period of milder subjective effects, followed by a return to normalcy.

The THC remaining in the blood undergoes two additional processes as it works its way through the body: treatment and disposal. Some reaches the liver, where a portion of it is chemically altered and rendered inert with each pass. As the circulatory system runs its cycle, more and more THC is deactivated and removed from the blood supply. Soon, the cannabinoid concentration in the blood drops below that in the brain and an osmotic exchange occurs in which the chemical flow reverses direction and moves THC from the brain back into the blood. The resinous effects diminish in the course of a few hours, as metabolites become inert and are redistributed more evenly throughout the body. Most accumulate in other fatty organs, particularly in *adipose* tissue—less politely known as common body fat. The inert compounds do not cause a high, but are sealed in fatty compounds and stored safely away with no further effect on the system. They accumulate in fat deposits at concentrations up to at least twenty times greater than in any other organ. The accumulation and removal of inert metabolites is particularly slow in the fat tissue, because blood flow to these depots is low. However, these processes steadily remove cannabinoids from the blood and transfer them to urine or fecal matter. The slow release of these stored inert substances results in the persistent appearance of THC metabolites in the urine for weeks after use of cannabis medicines.[14]

To study the metabolism and chemical transformation of THC in human subjects, researchers intravenously injected tracer doses of radiation-tagged THC into three subjects. Metabolites appeared in the bloodstream within ten minutes. Active levels in the plasma declined rapidly during the first hour after injection and more slowly thereafter. The researchers followed its course through blood, urine, and feces, and found that it was completely metabolized by the body. Negligible amounts of actual THC were excreted; instead, the metabolite 11-hydroxyl-Δ-9-THC appeared, along with cannabinol and other, more polar compounds.[15] The rapid decline in the first few hours probably represents metabolism and a redistribution of THC from the blood to body tissues, including the brain. This is followed by a slow decline over the next three days, which presumably represents retention and slow release from tissue stores. Over a period of eight days, 30 percent are excreted in the urine and 50 percent in the feces. Most are excreted in the first few days, and the remaining 20 percent are removed over the next seven or eight weeks. Various research reports have been published on drug testing, demonstrating that blood tests for cannabinoids are better indicators of resination than are urine tests, because cannabinoids in the blood are active, but the metabolites found in urine are inert.[16]

DEHYDRATION AND DIURETIC EFFECTS

We know that, as cannabis resin works its way through various body systems, it dries the mucus passages, the eyes, and the palate. Where does all that fluid go? It is used to flush out the system by increasing the flow of urine. This urine carries inert cannabinoid metabolites with it. Cannabis is a mild diuretic, as demonstrated by a study in which a healthy man was fed a diet for five days in which both the solids and liquids were kept constant in terms of quantity and kind. His urine was collected and measured while he was smoking cannabis on a daily basis, and a significant increase of urine output was demonstrated.

TOPICAL APPLICATIONS

Topical application means that a medicine is applied to the surface of the body rather than being consumed internally. A small amount may be dropped into the ear or rubbed into the skin, but the remedy is neither smoked nor eaten. For example, the flowers and leaves of the cannabis plant comprise a common topical folk remedy for the relief of swollen joints, inflammation, fever, infection, superficial injuries, burns, and rheumatism. In Mexico and Central America, cannabis leaves soaked in alcohol have traditionally been wrapped around aching, arthritic joints.

Czechoslovakian scientists discovered that the juicy resin pressed from flowering industrial hemp plants with ripe seeds, rich in CBD, is remarkably effective as an analgesic for burns and as an antibiotic against bacterial infections that might invade a wound or the ear, nose, and throat.[17] One researcher injured his thumb in the dissecting room and came down with an infection that was resistant to all available treatments. As amputation was being considered, his doctors decided to give the cannabis extract a try and found that it killed the infection, promoted healing, and saved the finger. The extract was also found to help control oral herpes and ulcerative gingivitis. Extracts of unripe cannabis tops demonstrated antibiotic activity against certain bacteria and fungi.[18] Bacteria-stopping and bacteria-killing properties have also been demonstrated in test tube studies that pit the cannabinoids against positive bacterial cultures.[19] CBD was found to be effective against strains of staphylococcus that were resistant to penicillin and other antibiotics.

Direct contact with THC killed herpes-virus lab cultures in a 1990 study at the University of South Florida.[20] There are anecdotal reports that a homemade alcohol-based tincture or poultice of cannabis can help clear up attacks of genital herpes, although the alcohol itself can be painful.

Ultimately it may turn out that the most beneficial aspect of using cannabis to treat some cancer may not be its ability to control pain, nausea, and sleeplessness, but a much more direct application. An experiment was conducted in the 1970s in which the lungs of mice were injected with cancer cells that grew into tumors. After Δ-9-THC, Δ-8-THC, or cannabinol was applied, the tumors shrank by 25 to 82 percent, depending on dose and duration of the treatment, with a corresponding increase in survival time.[21] Other animal studies also suggest that certain cannabinoids have tumor-reducing properties. Although there are no human studies to date, this could be a very exciting field of future research.

Ears

Cannabis has been used to treat maladies of the ears since antiquity. Two important Roman physicians of the second century A.D., Pliny the Elder and Galen, documented their use of cannabis to treat ear problems. The combination of antiseptic, anti-inflammatory, and analgesic effects of CBD and THC explains why, according to Galen, "Some squeeze its juice when fresh and use it as an analgesic for ear pains."

In England, the 1645 *Compleat Herbal* suggested using cannabis juice to eliminate "earwigs," an unpleasant affliction that was a problem for quite a long time. Culpeper's 1814 *Complete Herbal* agrees that the seeding flower is "Very good to kill the worms in men and beasts; and the juice dropped into the ears kills worms in them, and draws forth earwigs or other living creatures."

Warmed, but not hot, hempseed oil can be combined with ethyl alcohol, peroxide, and glycerine and dropped gently into the ear canal to soften ear wax and loosen hardened wax buildup. Shake just before using. Hold the patient's head at an angle to pour in the remedy, and let the oils saturate and soften the wax. After a few minutes, tilt the head back the other way to drain the ear, using a dropper to flush the ear canal with very warm water to remove the softened excess earwax. Repeat if necessary. This should be done every eight to twelve weeks to maintain the cleanliness of the ear.

Seed Oil Applications

The Greek historian Herodotus described Scythians in 450 B.C. using hemp to purify and cleanse themselves, which "makes their skin shining and clean."[22] Today, a growing number of hempseed-based personal hygiene products are on the market as soaps, shampoos, salves, cosmetics, and other skin and hair care items. A major area of research on essential fatty acids (EFAs) concerns their use in treating epidermal conditions such as psoriasis and eczema, marked by dry patches of raw or flaking skin. Direct application of EFAs has repeatedly demonstrated substantial improvement in skin smoothness, using both seed oils and omega-3-rich fish oils.[23] Since hempseed oil contains substantial amounts of omega-3, it is an excellent resource of oil for making therapeutic lotions and massage oils. The penetrating and replenishing nature of the oil on the skin also makes hempseed oil an excellent ingredient for lip balms to prevent chapping and dehydration, right down to the cellular level.

Hempseed is 30 to 35 percent oil, and a gallon of its oil weighs almost exactly eight pounds. In addition to foods, cooking oil, and dressings, industry uses this oil for making paints and varnishes, as well as ointments, lotions, and creams.[24] The importance of cleaning an injury with a good soap is well established, so hemp-based soaps have a direct medical utility. Adding CBD could produce antibiotic soaps. Cannabis medications can be applied directly to a cleaned wound, and even wrapped in hemp bandaging.

The Root of the Matter

Like ginger and ginseng, cannabis has a healthy root system that has proven beneficial to humanity. The *New English Dispensatory* of 1764 recommends boiling cannabis roots in water and directly applying the resulting paste to skin inflammations, both to soothe the injury and facilitate healing. The boiled root was also applied as a poultice to soothe joint pains and reduce inflammations. Another recommendation from about the same time period involved fresh hemp root crushed and mixed in butter to produce a topical cream that was applied to burns and abrasions.[25]

An important note of caution is due here. *The root is only suited for external use.* It is poisonous if consumed internally, and once figured in the political intrigues of medieval India.

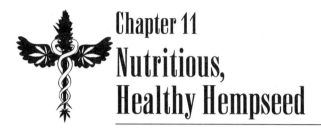

Chapter 11
Nutritious, Healthy Hempseed

The seed is the core of life and vitality. It transmits the DNA, reproduces the species, and nourishes the hemp seedling until the plant takes root in the nurturing earth and sends its tender shoot toward the heavens. Some suggest that the edible hempseed was discovered by our prehuman ancestors. Others, such as Carl Sagan, have contended that perhaps it was the very process of gathering and spilling hempseed around the seasonal campsites that led our nomadic forebears to invent agriculture, laying the foundation for the development of human culture and, thus, the birth of civilization.[1]

However it began, hempseed is a health-care product for the ages. The ancient Shinto priests used it in religious foods, such as *asanomi*. The National Institute of Oilseed Products told Congress in 1937 that hempseed "is used in all the Oriental nations and also in a part of Russia as food. It is grown in their fields and used as oatmeal. Millions of people every day are using hempseed in the Orient as food. They have been doing this for many generations, especially in periods of famine."[2] Drinking beverages made with boiled hempseed has been featured in the medical literature for millennia as a soothing remedy for coughs and throat irritations. Eating the seeds lubricates the

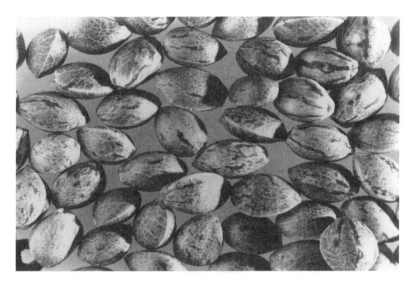

Hempseeds

bowels and is a traditional treatment for constipation, diarrhea, and digestive problems. Future investigations into the uses of hempseed oil's essential fatty acids are likely to look into many of the applications mentioned above, and to extend clinical research into arthritis, hypertension, diabetes, cancer, gastrointestinal disorders, ulcers, chronic fatigue syndrome, lupus, and more.

"Let food be your medicine. Let your medicine be your food," wrote Hippocrates. Yet the way food is selected and prepared has drastically changed over the past century. Food had traditionally been prepared in simple, seasonal combinations. Freshness was a primary concern. Today, foods are mechanically processed into complex combinations and treated with preservatives to increase shelf life and usability. Most Americans are deficient in trace minerals, vitamins, and essential fatty acids, but eat too much unhealthy fat, too few complex carbohydrates, too many empty calories, and too many unnecessary food additives. Hempseed is a tasty and healthy food item that fits comfortably into any diet regimen. It is a high-protein fruit

that contains a preferred nutritional ratio for bipeds, both human and bird. It provides a rare and valuable combination of
essential fatty acids that are now missing from most people's
daily eating routine. At the same time, the direct nutritional
use of hempseed is in resurgence. Rediscovered historical
records and new data are emerging that remind us of how important this seed oil is to our diet.

A broad range of symptoms that arise from linoleic acid
deficiency have recently been described by Udo Erasmus, including infections, impaired wound healing, retarded growth,
miscarriage, male sterility, skin eruptions, arthritic symptoms,
disturbed behavior, thirst with water loss through the skin, glandular dehydration, liver or kidney degeneration, cardiac problems, poor blood circulation, and hair loss.[3] Compare his list to
the recently translated uses of hempseed found in a four-hun-
dred-year-old medieval Chinese medical text, the *Pen T'sao Kang
Mu* (or *Ben Cao Gang Mu*).

> To mend and help all of the central areas, and benefit
> the *chi*. The Ancients used this medicine to remain fer-
> tile, strong and vigorous, and not be subject to aging. . . .
> It has the capacity to cure neurologic impairment due to
> stroke and the problems of excess sweating which it brings
> on. It has the power to cure dropsy and its accumulation
> of diluted lymph. It improves the urinary tract and the
> passing of urine. It can break up long-standing problems
> with the blood flow. It will restore the blood, the pulse,
> and the veins and arteries. It will alleviate retained pla-
> centa illness in mothers just beginning to suckle their
> infants. If one's head is washed with this, the hair will
> accelerate its growth, and be properly balanced with just
> the right amount of moisture.[4]

This great medical compendium of the Ming dynasty devoted
a major section exclusively to hempseed and its "calming" effect

on human physiology. It gives detailed recipes for hempseed remedies, and it is to these and other ancient formulas that the largest population on Earth owes much of its health. Clinical use of the cultivar *ma zi*, grown primarily for seed production, extends deep into the history of Chinese medicine. It was listed among the superior elixirs of immortality that are inherently nontoxic and can be taken for long or even indefinite periods of time. One variety of hemp, originally from Mao Luo Island in the Eastern Sea, was said to produce seeds of the "highest quality" that grew to the size of garden peas. This does not mean that everyone in China was having a psychoactive experience, however, since virtually all the plant's foliage was immediately composted to maintain soil quality.

EATING HEMPSEED

Hempseed is a primary food source that aids digestion. There are five general methods for preparing foods from hempseed: using whole seed, milling the seed, sprouting the seed, de-hulling the seed, and using the oil directly. When thoroughly cleaned, not even the most potent marijuana-type cannabis seed contains detectable amounts of the psychoactive chemical THC.[5] Cannabis plant lines that are grown for bearing the highest yields of hempseed are not selected to be high in THC content. Moreover, even the most resinous cannabis flower is shed by the plant as its seeds mature, and the dried remnants are simply brushed aside as the fruit is washed, prepared, and consumed. If properly cleaned, there is no residue left in the food item. Richard Rose, CEO of Sharon's Finest, explained what happened when his company introduced a hempseed-based cheese substitute called HempRella. "We had a Department of Justice lab in Oakland, California, test the product for THC, which they did and it was negative. They also ate some of it and the next day tested their urine for marijuana, and it too was negative. They felt that HempRella would not cause one to test positive for marijuana.

By extension one could say the hempseeds would also not cause one to test positive."

Hempseed is a versatile food item. Sprouting any raw seed improves its nutritional value. It also improves digestibility, increases the mass, and facilitates handling, since the hulls split and can be removed with water agitation. One pound of seed will yield three pounds of sprout. Even sterilized hempseed will sprout, although it will not germinate and grow into a viable plant. Hempseed sprouts can be used like any other seed sprout, in salads, stir-fries, or sandwiches. Like soybean, hempseed extracts can be made into vegetable milk, which mixes well nutritionally with soy milk. From soy milk one could make tofu, frozen dessert, cheese, or hundreds of other products. It can be solidified, texturized, and spiced to taste like chicken, beef, or pork. Hempseed can also be ground into meal, cooked like oatmeal or cream of wheat, then sweetened with milk, raisins, nuts, and dried fruits. Hempseed can be further ground into a margarine, common in Russia, that is similar to peanut butter but has a more delicate flavor. The seeds are roasted, seasoned, and eaten as a snack. Roasted and ground seeds can be baked into breads, cakes, pancakes, cookies, and casseroles. Some recipes appear later in this book.

If there is no THC in hempseed, what is in there? The Ohio Hempery had a lab assay done to find out. They learned that the seed is a combination of protein, carbohydrate, fatty acids, moisture, and ash. In combination, these provide dietary fiber, carotene, and a variety of vitamins, including B_1, B_2, B_3, B_6, C, and E. About 35 percent of the seed is dietary fiber, which includes most of the protein, all the ash, and some of the fatty acids. About 35 percent of the total seed is fatty acids in the form of a viscous oil. Another 25 percent is made up of amino acids, or protein.[6]

There are eight proteins that are essential to life that the human body cannot make, and two others which the body cannot make in sufficient quantity. These compounds must be con-

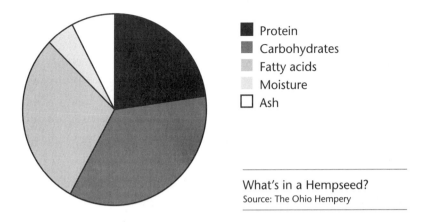

Protein
Carbohydrates
Fatty acids
Moisture
Ash

What's in a Hempseed?
Source: The Ohio Hempery

sumed in their natural form. The complete protein in hempseed gives the human body all the essential amino acids required to maintain health. It provides amino acids in the necessary types and amounts the body needs to make serum albumin and serum globulins, such as the immune-enhancing gamma globulin antibodies—the body's first line of defense.[7] Just a handful of hempseed provides this minimum daily nutrition for adults, and a bag full of it would provide all the essential protein, oils, and dietary fiber necessary for an adult to survive for two weeks, although it is unlikely to assuage their hunger.

The protein in hemp is more digestible than soy protein. Part of the reason for this is the presence of edestin. Hempseed protein is about 65 percent edestin, a sturdy protein that is pure, easy to prepare, and highly stable.[8] Edestin is so complete and nutritious that studies done in the early 1900s demonstrated that it could serve as the sole source of protein in the diet of animals.[9] The protein does not coagulate at room temperature, and is soluble in dilute salt solutions, unless it has been changed by a long period of exposure to heat. Unfortunately, federal law requires that all hempseed brought into the United States must be sterilized, and steaming is the most common method currently being used to destroy the seed's inner vitality. There are facilities around the country that receive the imported viable seed under customs bond, steam it at 212°F for 15 minutes, then issue a certificate of sterilization and release it to the consignee. This may slightly damage the edestin, making it less soluble in salt water and therefore less digestible. However, sterilized hempseed is still quite nutritious and people often roast or boil it before eating. This decision represents a trade-off between taste and benefit, but with hempseed—as with most vegetables—less cooking is better, nutritionally.

IN PURSUIT OF GOOD DIETARY FATS

We live in an age when the very idea of consuming fat is chastised and reviled. However, fats are a very concentrated source of energy and enhance the flavor of foods. It is important to recognize that, just like laws and people, there are good fats and there are bad fats. While overconsuming bad fats leads to obesity, cholesterol, and heart problems, consuming good fats helps ensure good health and a fortified immune system. The trick is knowing which is which.

Saturated fats, animal fats, and hydrogenated vegetable oils are bad fats. Essential fatty acid (EFA) is good fat. Raw hempseed oil is among the lowest in saturated fats, at just 8 percent of total oil volume. Instead, it has a lot of linoleic acid (LA), a type of EFA that is readily available in sesame, safflower, sunflower, and other commercial vegetable seed oils. LA, or omega-6, is related to oleic acid, linolenic acid (LNA), or omega-3, and gamma-linoleic acid (GLA). Researcher Lynn Osburn reports that "Hempseed is the highest in essential fatty acids of any plant. It contains all the essential amino acids and essential fatty acids needed to maintain healthy human life. No other single source provides complete protein in such an easily digestible form. No other plant has the oils essential to life in as perfect a ratio for human health and vitality." Hempseed oil content ranges from 51 to 62 percent LA, and from 19 to 25 percent LNA. Only flax oil has more linolenic acid, at 58 percent, but hempseed oil is still the highest in total essential fatty acid content, up to 81 percent of total oil volume.[10]

The exact proportion of individual EFAs in the seed is a variable. A nutritionally optimal three-to-one ratio of LA to LNA has been described for the long-term maintenance of good health. Hempseed oil contains anywhere from this ideal ratio down to about two-to-one. Dr. Andrew Weil, a long-time advocate of the use of flaxseed oil as a source of dietary EFA, found that hempseed has about 16 percent more total EFA than does flaxseed. Another advantage described by Weil is that hempseed oil has a good-tasting "nutty" flavor, whereas flaxseed oil made some of his patients gag. After two years of using flaxseed oil as a dietary supplement, researcher Udo Erasmus realized that he had developed "thin, papery-feeling skin that dried out and cracked easily." Other people developed similar conditions in as few as ten months of using only flaxseed oil. Erasmus attributed this to an imbalance caused by relying on flaxseed oil for his EFA supplement. Potential problems from long-term ingestion of oils like flaxseed, which are too rich in omega-3 LNA, might ultimately include symptoms such as inflammation in arthritis or immunosuppression. On review, Erasmus noted that hempseed, with its higher proportion of omega-6 LA, may hold nature's "most perfectly balanced oil."[11]

Gamma-linoleic acid (GLA), a particularly rare oil, is so beneficial to human growth and development that it is a component in the milk of nursing mothers. LNA has repeatedly been found effective in human studies for lowering cholesterol, but GLA is even more potent.[12] The body converts common LA into GLA by means of an enzyme, to protect itself from arthritis, premenstrual syndrome, and other conditions. Unfortunately, many factors in our diet can impair this ability, including the consumption of alcoholic beverages, processed vegetable oils, excess cholesterol, and heated cooking oils. In the decades since the suppression of industrial hemp cultivation, Americans have been

Percent of Fatty Acids in Health Oils[13]

	Hemp	Currant	Borage	Primrose	Flax
Linoleic (LA) (omega-6)	54.0	43.9	37.7	74.6	14
Linolenic (LNA) (omega-3)	21.1	14.5	4.3	—	58
G-Linoleic (GLA) (omega-3)	1.7	18.7	18.7	9.1	—

Sources: Udo Erasmus, Kenneth Jones, Andrew Weil.

able to obtain GLA only by consuming borage, black currant, or evening primrose seed oils to supplement their diet.[14] Today, hempseed is once again a readily available GLA source. Unfortunately, the oil is expensive due to the artificial economic restraint caused by the ban on producing domestic hemp.

CARING FOR YOUR HEMPSEED OIL

One problem associated with keeping a regular supply of hempseed oil is that it, like most high-quality vegetable oils, is structurally fragile. In the shell, seed oils endure for more than a year without major loss of nutritional value. However, hempseed oil's optimum refrigerated shelf life is less than two months after the seed has been pressed or the sealed container opened. Cold press is best suited for eating, while a hot press or chemical extraction may be appropriate for industrial applications. Food preparation affects nutritional quality, too. Cooking the delicate oil destroys much of its natural value. The smoke point of hempseed oil is 165°C, the flash point is 141°C, and the melting point is minus 8°C. Storing it too long at any temperature will result in its going rancid. Oil rancidity is a health risk. The measure of rancidity is how much peroxide and other toxic oxidation products have formed in the oil, called Peroxide Value (PV) and expressed as a number of milli-equivalents per kilogram. It usually should be less than 10 PV. Caution is advisable. An easy test that is fairly reliable is to smell the raw hempseed oil. It should have a mild aroma. If it has a very strong or bitter smell, or taste that bites the tongue, the oil should only be used for topical uses, such as massage.

Given the recent growth in the hempseed oil market, there may be new advances in maintaining freshness in the near future. In the meantime, to maximize the nutritional benefit and minimize risk of spoilage, use fresh oils taken by cold press, and use as little heat as possible in preparing foods. Keep the oil and the seeds out of sunlight, store in a cool, dark place, and don't wait too long to use it.

GOOD FOR CHILDREN
AND OTHER LIVING THINGS

We are living in a world of hunger. Some 75 percent of Central American children under the age of five are undernourished. A child dies every 2.3 seconds as a result of malnutrition, according to the UNICEF report, *State of the World's Children*. Some 38,000 children starve to death every day. Twenty million children die of malnutrition every year, according to the Institute for Food and Development Policy. The numbers are growing daily.

Wealthy nations, when they have done anything at all, temporarily ship grains from their food surplus. This does nothing to fix the problem. There's a better alternative to consider: give people a permanent food crop they can grow themselves. Hempseed can feed the hungry masses. It requires less attention than soy and less fuel to produce. It will grow in almost any climate where there is need, providing an easily obtained, high-quality source of protein.

Hempseed's nutritional benefits are not limited to humanity. It could also be used to feed poultry and livestock for a more ecologically sound base to the food chain. Even the "seed cake" left over from pressing the seed oil is edible—a virtually free source of animal feed derived from a crop that was raised for an entirely different purpose. Studies show that feeding hempseed to birds helps "bring back the feathers and improve the birds."[15] The seed is mixed with crushed, dried nettles and added to chicken feed during the winter to increase egg production.[16] As in the air, so in the water. "Fishes love this plant, and fly to it," wrote one Englishman, describing its use as bait.[17]

Apparently, no one can resist the healthy hempseed.

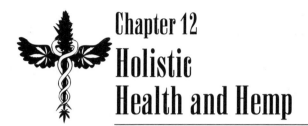

Chapter 12
Holistic
Health and Hemp

Most of the useful medicinal compounds in cannabis are not psychoactive, such as CBD and CBG. The federal government denies that they are active marijuana compounds because it officially recognizes THC as the only drug in cannabis. Hence, the others fall into a category of hemp products that are not technically marijuana. Three other health factors fall outside the definition of marijuana, too: nutrition, hygiene, and environment. Hempseed is important to maintaining proper nutritional balance and to bolstering the immune system. Hemp gives us antibacterial compounds and cleaning agents. Hemp fiber offers critical medical supplies such as slings and bandaging. But the economic and ecological benefits rising from the large-scale development of industrial hemp may ultimately prove to be this plant's greatest gift to health—individual, societal, even planetary. Wildlife consume hempseed, and the growing plants add air to the soil and oxygen to the air, so simply sowing cannabis and letting it grow wild is a good way to help the planet. Consider, then, the holistic health benefits of fully developing industrial hemp as a restorative natural resource.

ENVIRONMENT AFFECTS HEALTH

Nature has been the proverbial "canary in the coal mine" for humanity since the industrial revolution hit in the early eighteenth century. It takes simple common sense to recognize that if a chemical kills bugs, plants, and animal pests, it probably kills people, too. Chief Seattle gave his ominous warning to the United States Congress in 1854: "Whatever befalls the earth befalls the sons of the earth. Man did not weave the web of life. He is merely a strand in it. Whatever he does to the web, he does to himself." Each new life form that is lost, estimated at one thousand species per year, and each local ecosystem that is destroyed gives another warning that we are in a global environmental crisis. The subtle interconnections of planetary chemistry and personal well-being make it difficult to pinpoint a simple cause for the complex syndrome of health problems that arise from a deteriorated environment. However, ample direct linkages have been established over the years, such as cancers caused by pesticides and toxic wastes.

Frogs in Minnesota, Wisconsin, South Dakota, and even as far away as Vermont and Quebec, Canada, have recently shown an alarming rise in mutations and deformities. Researchers suspect that the cause is some sort of water pollution caused by airborne contaminants, possibly including pesticides and heavy metals. The implication for human populations is frightening, also. In the wetland where the anomalies were first noticed in large numbers, virtually every household has at least one cancer patient, according to the local middle-school teacher whose biology students made the initial discovery.[1]

God will "destroy them which destroy the earth," says the Bible. But the human race may be saving God the trouble by destroying itself. It is no exaggeration to say that our modern ecological crisis is a health crisis of epic proportions, and our ability to solve environmental problems will determine our survival as a society, and as a species. It is time to reassess and redirect our activities, before it is altogether too late.

SUSTAINABLE INDUSTRY

Most of our basic raw materials used for home and industry today come from mining, drilling, and forestry. Using farm crops to make the same products means that we can finally stop destroying our environment, if we use the right crops and manufacturing technologies. This brings us back to industrial hemp. Developing a sustainable domestic resource with the versatility of hemp assures a consistent and stable economy with the flexibility to encounter changing circumstances.

A resource is sustainable when it can renew itself as quickly as we consume it. Hemp grows for a few months and dies at the end of its season, whether harvested or not, leaving its seed, stalk, and fiber behind. The next year, it grows right back. Our industries can keep using hemp year after year, and our farms will grow it year after year. As demand grows, simply plant more hemp. Hemp grows abundantly here. It lends itself to a wide variety of methods and circumstances of manufacture, from cottage industries to mass production. Hemp is one of the most profitable agricultural crops to grow, and among the easiest industrial feedstocks to use.[2] It can be manufactured to produce food, clothing, housing, paper, plastic, energy, and many other essential consumer goods. Henry Ford built a car using hemp in 1941, and Daimler Benz hopes to do the same in 1997.[3] Where equipment is scarce but labor is plentiful, hemp can be worked by hand on a small scale. It is possible to build new equipment and factories, or to adapt and retrofit existing industrial facilities for modified production. The changeover of technology is a normal process of attrition for business, as old equipment wears out and is replaced.

Sustainability provides better job security. For example, the work of most timber-related jobs does not consist of chopping down trees, but of the transportation, milling, distribution, marketing, sale, and use of timber industry end products in the form of construction materials and paper. Hemp production can rapidly expand to a level that will help maintain and expand these commercial activities. A strong argument can be made for getting big government out of the hemp business and letting the private sector determine the course of investment and development.[4]

Harvesting an annual crop to build a house that will stand for fifty or one hundred years is highly sustainable. Cutting down a five-hundred-year-old tree to publish a daily newspaper is not the least bit sustainable. The U.S. Department of Agriculture already knew this in 1916, when it produced *Bulletin 404,* reporting that our forests were being cut down three times faster than they grew. It called for alternatives to the use of timber and recommended using hemp pulp for paper instead of tree pulp. Over twenty years, hemp will produce four times as much pulp per acre as will forest land.[5] Since hemp is a seasonal crop, it could most practically be used to extend the supply of other natural resources, such as using hemp in the fall and winter and shifting to tree farms in the spring and summer. That would assure a continuous, year-round supply of raw material.

In addition to its nutritional and topical therapeutic uses described earlier in this book, hempseed has many industrial uses. These include soap, paint, fuel and heating oil, precision engine lubricants, varnish, lacquer, sealants, plastics, and so on. Historically, the domestic demand has almost always exceeded the supply that was produced by American farms, and so industry has relied on imports from China, Russia, and other lands. The U.S. imported 116 million pounds of hempseed in 1935 alone.[6] A lot of that went into paints, because hempseed oil is a good drying agent. The Sherwin Williams Paint Company's famous "cover the world" logo showed the planet being covered with hempseed-oil–based paints until the 1937 ban forced the company to switch to petroleum and lead-based paints.[7] It could now be time for them to switch back.

RESTORATIVE AGRICULTURE

Farms always need a profitable crop, and hemp is an ideal one. Hemp is a hardy, pest resistant, soil-building plant that is excellent in crop rotation. Hemp patches have played important roles in erosion control, reforestation, weed eradication, supporting wildlife habitat, and reducing air and water pollution. The plant's strong roots anchor and aerate the soil to control erosion and mud slides. This is especially beneficial in recently deforested areas. It grows best in warm tropical zones or moderately cool, temperate climates. Hemp seedlings endure cold or light frost as well as oat seedlings or other spring crops. Certain strains of this traditional cash crop do quite well in mild droughts, thanks to the plant's deep tap root.[8] Hemp plants shed their leaves throughout the growing season, adding rich organic matter to the topsoil. Hemp crops never need chemical herbicides and rarely need any pesticides.[9] In fact, the plant has so few serious insect enemies that it is said to have been used to make organic pest repellents.[10] It is often possible to grow two crops in the same year. The best fertilizer for hemp is manure applied to the preceding crop. Hemp is sown as "green fertilizer" to prepare the ground for the next crop. It can be grown on muck lands for purposes other than fiber.[11] Hemp squeezes out weeds, and leaves the soil in excellent condition for any succeeding crop, especially when weeds may otherwise be troublesome.[12]

Farmers reported excellent hemp growth for nearly one hundred years on land that was steadily cultivated. Yields can easily come in at three to five tons of stalk per acre, including about a ton of nature's finest natural fiber for textiles and high density composites, plus more than a ton of cellulose for paper and construction material, plus plenty of leftovers for compost, fuel, or plastics. Factor in the seed's economic potential, and it's clear that a farm can turn a decent profit.

The agricultural community has begun to recognize this fact. The first industrial hemp bill was introduced into the New York legislature by Senator Joe Galiber. Delegates to the 1996 national convention of the American Farm Bureau Federation voted overwhelmingly in favor of research into reviving domestic industrial hemp development. The Kentucky Bourbon County Farm

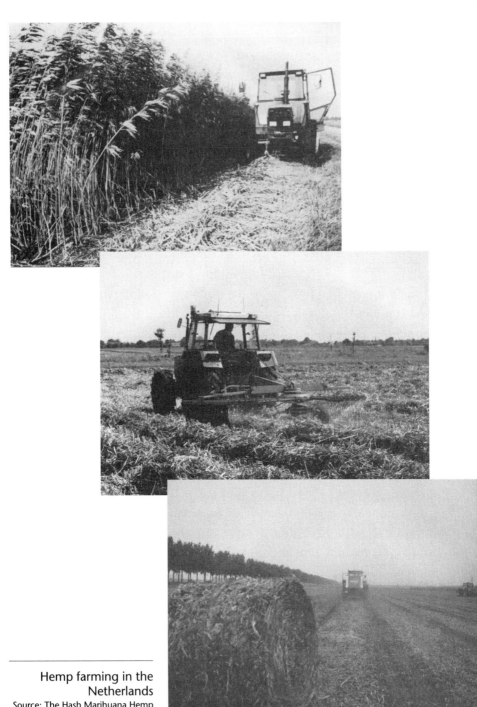

Hemp farming in the
Netherlands
Source: The Hash Marihuana Hemp
Museum

Bureau passed a follow-up Industrial Hemp Resolution on October 10, 1996, stating, "We support the development of industrial hemp (by definition less than 1 percent THC) and urge the Farm Bureau to put its full resources into getting the laws changed to allow this." Legislation authorizing research into restoring industrial hemp was adopted in two states at opposite ends of the country in 1996, Vermont and Hawaii, and attempted in two others, Colorado and Missouri. As the traditional southern and midwestern hemp belt takes renewed interest in hemp, pressure for legislative reform is likely to mount. So far the federal government has not allowed any field tests to proceed. Obviously, the key to the whole process of agriculture is to get the seed into the soil, and let commerce grow from there.

HEALING THE EARTH

It's called earth, but we treat it like dirt. Soil is a precious but unappreciated resource. Loss of topsoil has been a plague throughout the ages, and has caused many great civilizations to fall. The fields of Europe and Asia have been tilled for millennia. The world has supported agriculture for over ten thousand years.

The New World was legendary in Europe for its fertile soil. Thomas Morton attributed the fact that hemp in New England grew twice as high as that in England to the richness of the soil.[13] Thomas Paine felt that America was ripe for revolution because the hemp harvest was flourishing and abundant enough to outfit a Continental army and navy.[14] Thomas Jefferson and Gouverneur Morris urged farmers in 1791 to stop growing tobacco and return to hemp, which is easier on the soil, because "a material for manufactures of various sorts, becomes afterwards the means of support to numbers of people, hence it is to be preferred in a populous country." Hemp covered the wagons and powered the sailing ships that expanded the nation and brought great wealth and trade.

But times changed. Severe restrictions were placed on growing hemp early this century in the U.S. Soon major droughts
hit, and the midwestern farm states were dubbed "the dust bowl."
The wind which had hung heavy with hemp pollen and the water which had run clear were thick and brown with the topsoil
they carried away. The region's farm economy was destroyed
and the environment has still never fully recovered. Over two-
thirds of our original topsoil was lost between the beginning of
European colonization and the late 1980s.[15] Current loss of agricultural land here continues at over five billion tons per year.[16]
Some of this is caused by logging forests, but 85 percent results
from croplands, pastures, range land, and forest land directly
used for raising cattle and other livestock.[17] Something is dread-
fully wrong when centuries of topsoil are consumed in a few
generations.

SAVING THE TREES

They are the lungs of the planet, and they're being eaten away
every day. Over 97 percent of our American forests have been
destroyed under the relentless onslaught of economic expan-
sion. In 1988 alone, 226 million tons of trees were pulped for
paper. Today 93 percent of the world's paper is made from trees.
If forestry practices were truly sustainable, we would not have
needed to log any virgin forests for decades now, yet the devasta-
tion goes on. The battle to save the world's last remaining virgin
redwood forests in California from logging interests highlights
the falsehood of the claim that forests are a renewable resource.
Even as logging companies claim that their monoculture tree
farms can meet the demand, they also say they need to "harvest"
most of the remaining natural mixed-growth forests. Someone
is lying, and nature is dying.

Forests protect and nurture the diversity of life on the planet.
When we lose the forests, we lose a lot more than precious trees.
We lose entire ecosystems that are built around them. We kill off

entire species with impunity. As many as one-fourth of all mammal species are now described as "endangered," meaning that they are at imminent risk of extinction. That includes one-half of all monkeys and apes, according to the World Conservation Union, which has conducted an annual study for more than thirty-five years. The project evaluated the chances of survival for all 4,025 known species of mammals, and it does not look good. "If anything, we've been too optimistic" in previous assessments of the health of biodiversity, noted primate specialist Russell Mittermeier.[18]

This situation is due in part to pollution and in part to the introduction of non-native species into established ecological systems. The bigger part of the problem is the destruction and fragmentation of wildlife habitat, which causes the other two problems. This is a consequence of the expansive nature of our economic development. Rainforests are often logged or burned down simply to clear more land for grazing and farming. The topsoil soon washes away, and the land becomes barren, so the slash and burn process moves to devour its next morsel of land. What the world needs is an emergency dose of hemp in all agricultural regions. Since traditional hemp agriculture does not wear out soil, the land retains its fertility, and there is no need to clear more forest.

Each ton of paper made from hemp saves twelve mature trees. Hemp and trees are both made of wood, but because cannabis is an annual plant, it constructs a less durable organic structure than a tree requires to stand for decades and longer. Paper made from hemp requires substantially less of the acids and other toxic chemicals used to break trees down into pulp. Because the bast fiber of hemp is so much longer than the wood fiber of trees, paper made with hemp can be recycled more than twice as many times as tree-pulp paper before losing its strength. Hemp can also be made into fiberboard, particle board, or variable density composite boards for all types of mold making, construction, and commercial fabrication. In other words, anything now made with trees can be made with hemp. We can continue to have paper, build homes and other structures, expand our productivity, and still let our forests grow and breathe.

Unfortunately, the trees keep falling, and as the forest goes, so goes much of its inherent moisture. Certain strains of hemp grow well in dryer conditions, such as those that follow the loss of forest canopy.[19] Tight rows of hemp, planted in a wide belt hugging the tree line, form a wind block to help maintain the natural humidity within the standing groves and hold weeds at bay while the damaged forest recovers. Theoretically, a systematic planting of hemp along the edges of man-made deserts in the course of coming decades could eventually return them to marginal land, then crop land, and finally, back to forest.

WATER, AIR, AND ENERGY

Water is nature's way of flushing and refreshing Earth's lifeforms. Chemical water pollution has a catastrophic effect on the environment, but also directly on people's health, and has been linked to numerous cancers and birth defects.[20] In the U.S. alone, agricultural pollution, including soil, fertilizer, and pesticide runoff, accounts for more pollution than all municipal and industrial sources combined.[21] We can reduce this problem at its source. Cotton, corn, sugar cane, and tobacco are among the hardest crops on the soil, in terms of chemical applications and nutrient depletion. They all require heavy fertilization. While it is possible to grow quality organic cotton, in general cotton is the most chemical-intensive crop ever grown. It uses a lot of water and about seventeen separate applications of fungicides, herbicides, pesticides, and defoliants in the course of its growing cycle. About half of all agriculture chemicals are used on cotton.[22] Yet, an acre of land will produce two or three times as much hemp fiber as cotton and serve all the same industrial uses, plus certain high-tech applications for which cotton is unsuited.

Livestock in the U.S. produces 230,000 pounds of excrement

each and every second, much of which ends up as runoff water pollution. Fortunately, this is actually the best possible natural fertilizer for hemp, which digests the manure and simultaneously controls both erosion and chemical runoff. By switching from crops that require massive doses of chemical fertilizers to crops like hemp that prefer to consume the manure oversupply, we can solve several problems at once and have an overall increase of productivity.

Rivers might be characterized as the bloodstream of the planet; the beverage from which most land species drink their life. These rivers feed our lakes and reservoirs, and serve as the direct water supply for communities everywhere. Pulp mills kill rivers with foul-smelling and poisonous effluence. As raw material for pulp and paper, hemp can greatly reduce the mills' use of sulfur-based acids that are used to break down tree cellulose, a major source of river contamination. This means less water pollution from the timber pulping process. Tree-free hemp paper can be made without dioxin-producing chlorine bleach, another toxin in both our water and our air. The federal EPA estimates that 99 percent of airborne dioxin emissions come from incineration of medical and municipal waste that contains chlorine.[23] Much of this comes from papers and fabrics that have been bleached to create an impression of cleanliness and purity. The consequences of all this whiteness have been dire, indeed, for the planet and its inhabitants. Atmospheric ozone acts as a shield against ultraviolet radiation—a shield that chlorine is rapidly disintegrating. The hole in the ozone layer is now over 8.5 million square miles, twice the area of Europe's landmass. The increased radiation is already causing skin carcinomas among sunbathers and cataract blindness in wildlife, particularly in the Southern hemisphere. An update report to the 1996 United Nations conference on ozone depletion estimated that the ozone layer could be depleted by 40 percent by the year 2075, causing an additional 154 million cases of skin cancer and 3.4 million more deaths in the U.S. alone.[24]

The earth not only has a hole in its halo, it has a bad case of gas, too. There has been an alarming increase in the amount of "greenhouse gas" in the atmosphere. Carbon dioxide (CO_2) is a gas that the atmosphere holds in place like the windows of a greenhouse, capturing heat that is normally reflected back into space. This pollution buildup is a direct result of burning, mostly of fossil fuels like petroleum and coal. Many experts consider this chemical imbalance to be a key factor in regional weather changes and global warming, possibly leading to desertification. Other effluents from burning fossil fuels include carbon monoxide, a carcinogen, as well as sulfur dioxide and nitrous oxide, two components of acid rain. Both individually and in combination, these pollutants cause lung disorders and significant ecological harm. The situation is eerily reminiscent of a warning given by Mohammed in the Koran, "The heaven shall produce a visible smoke, which shall cover mankind; this will be a tormenting plague." This degradation is often characterized as an unavoidable consequence of the economy-versus-ecology tradeoff. Contrary to opinion, however, the condition is treatable.

Nature has devised an effective system to clean the air. Rainfall pulls down dust and particulate matter. Plant photosynthesis converts CO_2 back into oxygen. Growing plants take the CO_2, remove the carbon atom and use it to build carbohydrate vegetable matter, then release the leftover oxygen into the air. Biofuel technology can convert plant matter into a wide range of fuels and energy. Hemp produces a larger amount of dry vegetable matter than almost any other rotational farm crop suited for temperate climates.[25] Each crop produces as much oxygen while growing as it produces CO_2 if burned as fuel, creating a balanced cycle. Furthermore, hemp deposits 10 percent of its mass in the soil as roots and up to 30 percent as leaves that drop throughout the growing season. This means that some 20 to 40 percent more oxygen can typically be produced each season than will be polluted—a net gain in clean air, for a "reverse greenhouse effect."

When the sky cries, it must really be hurting. Acid rain hits when certain contaminants have a chemical reaction as they wash out of the air. Fossil fuels contain sulfur, and when burned they form air pollution containing sulfur dioxide (SO_2). When SO_2 combines with rain water (H_2O), they form sulfurous acid (H_2SO_3). This common form of acid rain eats away at our fields, forests, cars, buildings, and monuments. Trees and other plants, lakes and rivers are damaged first by the liquid acid and then by the resulting soil-chemistry imbalances. The buildup of acids in our lakes and ponds is thought to be a major factor behind the precipitous reduction of amphibians globally.[26]

Biofuels do not contain sulfur or lead unless they are intentionally added, which is not necessary. Hemp makes an excellent biofuel source. It can be grown as an energy crop, or fuel could be produced from its waste material left over from manufacturing textile, paper, or other consumer goods. During the Second World War, the head of the U.S. War Hemp Industries Corporation explained that hemp waste was burned to power its own mills, potentially generating a huge energy surplus.[27] "Fiber is obtained from the stems of the plant, *Cannabis sativa.* All of the factories use the hurd to fire the huge boilers which provide heat for drying and power to operate the machines. Fuel costs are eliminated through this ingenious procedure." This power can be profitably sold back to the utility companies to feed the overall energy grid.

Perhaps use of hemp as a combustible fuel will turn out to be a transition into even cleaner technologies, like photovoltaic cells and hydrogen fuel. Until that day, we still need cleaner fuel. The most hazardous toxic wastes arise from two industries, petrochemicals and nuclear power. Hemp and other biofuels can safely, cleanly, and significantly reduce the use of these destructive resources. We will still need to refine, transport, and store finished fuel for use, creating some level of accident risk, but many important advantages remain. Less reliance on petroleum means fewer oil wells, fewer oil well fires, and fewer oil spills to destroy marine life, birds, and beaches. A hemp spill is relatively harmless and easy to clean up. Similarly, without nuclear reactors there will be no nuclear utility accidents, no radioactive waste, leaks, or spills, and no danger of terrorist attacks. In terms of national security, nuclear reactors and oil fields are tempting military targets; bombing hemp fields would be rather ineffective. The economic arguments for nuclear power and fossil fuels fall apart in light of the massive subsidies needed, such as military costs of protecting oil fields, cleanup costs, and the health costs borne by society. Department of Energy estimates suggest that renewable energy plus conservation could produce a return on investment of almost $100 for every dollar spent, through avoided oil imports and environmental damage.[28]

OTHER ECO-CONSIDERATIONS

The way that we eat can change the world, and the American diet has changed radically in recent decades. By 1985 Americans ate only half as much grains and potatoes as in 1909. Consumption of beef soared by almost half. Poultry consumption nearly tripled. This had an important effect on seemingly unrelated areas of the economy and environment. Livestock consume grain and other food items, and require additional equipment and health care. The cumulative energy value used to produce one calorie of beef protein is 78 calories of fuel, while one calorie of soybean protein takes only two calories of fuel.[29] If Americans reduced their intake of meat by just 10 percent, an estimated 100 million people could be adequately nourished using the land, water, and energy freed from growing livestock feed.[30] Nutritious hempseed serves as food, as vegetable oil and, if necessary, as fuel oil. Properly processed, even the hemp stalk offers a plentiful source of dietary fiber.

There's another good reason to consider changing livestock production patterns, too. In 1960, 13 percent of staphylococci infections were penicillin-resistant; in 1988 it was 91 percent. Why are germs becoming increasingly immune to drugs? Many people think it is simply due to overuse. About 55 percent of antibiotics used in the U.S. are fed routinely to livestock, with or without signs of illness.[31] United States meat and pharmaceutical industries support this practice. The European Community bans it because they suspect it acts as a natural selection process, killing off the weaker germs while allowing drug-resistant germs to multiply, flourish, and dominate the gene pool. In other words, survival of the fittest germs, which is bad news for the rest of us. Feeding our livestock hempseed is a way to support their immune systems and bolster the animals' overall health without using antibiotics until their use is necessary and justifiable. Animals fed hempseed could prove to be healthier and more disease-resistant, but since the mechanism is nutritional rather than antibiotic, bacteria would not become resistant.

Hemp's role as a restorative resource is evident in its horticultural uses. Growing hemp can extract heavy metal contaminants from the chemically degraded soil in damaged farm lands, so the lands can again be used for growing food crops. Researchers in Poland experimenting with this process are having good results. This does not eliminate the toxins, it merely draws them from the soil and fixes them into the fiber of the hemp plants, which are then used to make non-edible items. This is safer than having them in the food supply, but the toxins still end up at disposal sites when the end product is finally discarded. The researchers are looking for a way to extract the toxins from the fiber to solve this dilemma and dispose of them properly. The net effect could be to create a supply of recycled heavy metals for industrial applications.[32]

While important industrial crops like the loblolly pine, used for paper, and the soybean, used for food, face a potential 30 to 50 percent loss in productivity from increased ultraviolet radiation due to ozone depletion, the hemp plant remains largely unfazed. Cannabis merely increases its output of resinous cannabinoids, which seem to provide a shield, and keeps right on growing.[33] To better ensure survival of the species, when its seeds are exposed to high levels of ultraviolet light hemp increases its output ratio of female to male plants.[34] Hemp will thus offer a continuing source of raw material for consumer goods, long after other sources begin to die off from radiation. This will protect both our productivity and jobs until the problem is properly solved, which may well take centuries.

Returning from plastics to natural fiber will reduce the buildup of solid waste that threatens to bury our society. In a few situations, ultra-lightweight plastic rope may be preferable, but a good, strong, biodegradable hemp rope will still meet most cordage needs. Plastic bags can largely be eliminated and replaced with reusable cloth or recyclable paper bags made of tree-free hemp cellulose. Hemp cardboard packaging can be designed to replace most Styrofoam containers. Another critical advantage of returning to hemp as an industrial feed stock is the job-intensive nature of its use, allowing more people to afford healthier lives. There are jobs on the farm to prepare the soil, plant, and harvest the crop. There are transportation jobs to move it to the mill. There are jobs at the mill for preliminary processing, and the product is then transported to the factory for finishing. By now the commodities market and stock market are starting to get their value out of the crop. After inspection, the goods are shipped to the distributor, who sells it to the wholesaler, who puts it onto the retail market. The ordering departments, inventory control, and clerical staff get ready to move the goods to the public. Once purchased, many items like paper and building supplies go on to be used in other trades and businesses, creating even more job opportunities.

The rebounding hemp industry is evident in international symposia and conferences like Germany's 1995 *Biofach* and 1996 *Europhalle CannaBusiness Expo*. Entrepreneurs and investors have created new companies and joined together to form the Hemp Industries Association (HIA) to protect their interests and the integrity of the trades.[35] Economic opportunity relieves a lot of personal stress, and that's healthy, too.

Restoring hemp will allow future generations to breathe cleaner air, drink cleaner water, and enjoy cleaner environs with healthier lakes, rivers, and forests to enjoy. This planet can still be the garden paradise we deserve—a beautiful, bountiful world. Society needs forests and quiet spaces where we can ponder life and draw strength. But we need to be better gardeners.

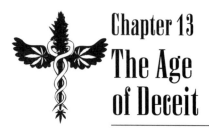

Chapter 13
The Age
of Deceit

A rational soul might think it pointlessly cruel for a wealthy nation to provide no health care for the vast majority of its citizens, then proceed to inflict criminal penalties upon sick and dying people who use a medicine that is not officially authorized, yet that is exactly what happens. Left to their own desperate resources, millions of Americans find that medical relief can be grown for free in their own home garden, in the form of a few lush cannabis plants. At some point, it becomes worth it to pay almost any price or run any risk, simply to get relief. Many choose to run that risk in hopes of being cured before being arrested. Then the enforcement trap is sprung; the drug task force kicks in the door, knocks in walls, grabs all the money, rounds up the family on the ground with automatic weapons aimed at their heads, and begins asking who wants to testify against whom, in exchange for a lighter sentence. The harm done to patients by criminal prosecution and punishment greatly exceeds any possible harm these people might cause by even their wildest excessive misuse of cannabis. In many cases, criminal penalties rival the consequences of even the most horrible physical maladies that afflict these patients.

But that's the difference between rationality and rationalizations. Unfortunately, we live in an age of deceit. Federal agencies of the United States rely on disinformation and brute force to prevail over the face of logic and human decency. They trot out spin doctors to explain why taxpayers must continue to foot the bill for a failed policy that is such a sacred cow politicians are afraid to even discuss it. They pull out smoke and mirrors to dazzle us with their propagandistic aplomb. Then they throw up a cloud of scientific dust into our eyes to keep us from seeing their hidden agendas. Pity the poor deceivers when their mask of respectability is pulled away from them, and their true motivations stand exposed.

PROTECTING THE PUBLIC FROM THE TRUTH

Marijuana is not a "cure all." No drug is. In fact, marijuana does not cure much of anything; it merely helps to relieve and control specific symptoms—lots of different symptoms, some worse than others, scattered throughout the incredibly complex human anatomy. Like a panacea, it is very broad in scope, and can alleviate suffering for millions of Americans.

The public is not supposed to know that, and must therefore be protected from the facts. John Ingersoll, the first Director of the federal Drug Enforcement Administration (DEA), put it this way in 1972: "Not only are we here to protect the public from vicious criminals in the street but also to protect the public from harmful ideas."[1] He promptly set about fabricating an exciting sideshow of "new" and "scientific" myths, such as unproved theories about brain damage, cancers, lab cultures jumping through hoops, uncontrollable weight gain, and the ever-amazing "pot grows breasts on men." That last claim got a lot of transsexuals' hopes up and set them to smoking like chimneys, but with little success.

After ten years, the Institute of Medicine finally reviewed the rumors of "new dangers" of marijuana in 1982 and released a study that contradicted most of the claims. The report found that no solid evidence of adverse effects from moderate use of cannabis had been demonstrated. Then the tax-exempt Partnership for a Drug Free America (PDFA) began a commercially polished, mass media propaganda blitz defaming productive members of society who smoked marijuana, forcing many into denial, and sometimes turning their children against them. The tragedy is that this carefully orchestrated campaign is built upon the legitimate concerns of unsuspecting parents, physicians, and social scientists who don't know the facts needed to see through the absurd misrepresentations of the generally benign and helpful nature of the plant *Cannabis sativa* L.

Not until 1995 did the world's preeminent scientific journal, *Lancet*, again review the data and conclude that "The smoking of cannabis, even long term, is not harmful to health."[2] Dr. James Spurlock summarized the situation on marijuana as, "Medical researchers know it's a pharmacological substance which can do great good."[3] However, the American Medical Association says it cannot endorse medical marijuana until approved controlled studies are completed. That makes sense. But millions of patients go on suffering, or self-medicate and take the risk that their lives and reputations will be destroyed by law enforcement, while we wait on those studies. Science should guide politics, not vice versa. Yet, we see over and over the steadfast perversion of published findings and statistics designed to give the drug warriors what they need to stay in business.

It is not within the scope of this book to elaborate the details of this corrupting system, so instead I devote a few pages to a review of the more egregious errors, misrepresentations, and overgeneralizations propagated by the drug warriors.

YOUR BRAIN ON EGGS

No marijuana scare campaign has ever been complete without bringing up brain damage. And no claim of cannabis causing physical brain damage has ever been proven. The primary basis for this fear was the Heath Monkey study. Dr. Robert Heath's research alleging brain damage from smoking cannabis was met with widespread skepticism from the start, because it contradicted previous findings. The initial peer review warned that Heath's claims "must be interpreted with caution. . . . No definitive interpretation can be made at this time." Closer examination revealed that basic lab procedures regarding tissue preparation, fixation, and photography had not followed proper controls or safeguards against contamination and bias. The monkeys were forced to inhale immense amounts of cannabis smoke through oxygen masks for long periods of time, with no opportunity to breathe fresh air. The tissue damage Heath documented was indicative of oxygen deprivation. Once this was factored into the equation, cannabis was ruled out as a significant factor in the tissue damage. Repeated follow-up studies still cannot document significant brain tissue problems associated with marijuana.

Curiously, Heath's monkey experiment had been carried out more professionally some eighty years earlier. In 1892, the Raj Commission conducted a clinical experiment in which a rhesus monkey took 181 inhalations of ganja smoke over a period of eight months and ten days, at a daily dosage proportional to a heavy smoker. After sacrificing the animal, a meticulous autopsy found "no evidence of any brain lesions being directly caused by hemp drugs. There is evidence that the coarse brain lesions produced by alcohol and dhatura are not produced by hemp drugs."

The classic PDFA ad is a picture of an egg in its shell, labeled "Your brain." The next picture is a fried egg in a skillet, labeled "Your brain on drugs." Followed by "Any questions?" Actually, yes. For starters, what does an egg in a skillet really have to do with my brain? More importantly, why do the alcohol, tobacco, and pharmaceutical drug industries, all of which produce products that cause physical brain damage, contribute so much tax-deductible money to produce ads that trick people into thinking cannabis does?

SMOKING MEDICINE

Opening up the *British Medical Journal* of Nov. 11, 1897, we read, "Hemp therefore exerts its effects differently according to the preparation used. . . . In cases where an immediate effect is desired, the drug should be smoked, the fumes being drawn through water. In fits of depression, mental fatigue, nervous headache, and exhaustion, a few inhalations produce an almost immediate effect, the sense of depression, headache, feeling of fatigue disappear and the subject is enabled to continue his work, feeling refreshed and soothed. I am further convinced that its results are marvelous in giving staying power and altering the feelings of muscular fatigue which follow hard physical labour."[4]

In 1980 cancer patients demonstrated clear benefits from smoked marijuana, and their preference for smoking it was again established in 1987 in the Vinciguerra study.[5] Dozens of cannabis buyers clubs have provided smoking material for thousands of patients in the 1990s. A majority of oncologists responding to a Harvard University survey in 1991 agreed that they should be allowed to prescribe it.[6] Legislators in thirty-seven states have endorsed medical marijuana, and voters in Arizona and California approved its use by margins of more than 10 percentage points in 1996.

In other words, resinous cannabis has always been and will continue to be smoked as medicine. In fact, it is being smoked right now, in your home town, for medicinal purposes.

THE LUNG'S FAIR SHARE

Is marijuana four times as dangerous as tobacco or a zillion times more so? It all depends on which tobacco lobbyist you ask. Proponents of this claim point to smokers' intake of two specific items—smoke particulate and carbon monoxide—and only in the large air passage of the lungs. If you ignore everything else, greater concentrations do occur in marijuana smoke, and it does

Photo: Rev. Hemp

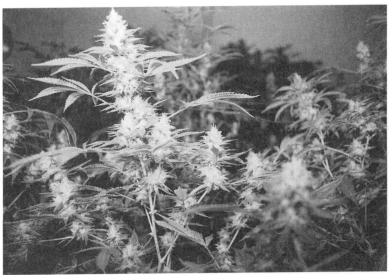

Grow room for a Texas buyers club.

cause lesions in that one air passage. These lesions are described as "precancerous" in press reports about marijuana, although scientists admit they have no proof that the lesions lead to cancer. Yes, this is cause for minor concern, and cannabis smoking could contribute to bronchitis. But put this in perspective. Cigarette smokers are measured by how many packs-a-day they consume. There are 400,000 deaths a year attributed to tobacco, many of them extremely painful due to gruesome lung cancers. Addicted patients suck on cigarettes as their last breath slips away.

Zero deaths a year are attributed to the direct physical effect of consuming marijuana. In fact, Miles Herkenham, a brain researcher at the National Institute of Mental Health, says that "It's impossible to take a lethal overdose. You absolutely cannot kill an animal with THC."[7] Cannabis smoke does irritate the lungs a bit, but almost nobody chain-smokes marijuana. It's usually a matter of a few puffs on the weekend or up to several joints per day as a medical dosage.

This brings up one of the best kept secrets about cannabis.

The active compounds are assimilated almost instantly when smoke is taken into the lungs. After a few seconds, the ratio of beneficial to potentially destructive compounds in the smoke takes a negative turn. In other words, holding the smoke in longer doesn't increase THC intake as much as it increases the health risk. The government has known this since at least 1970, but is so eager to produce evidence of lung damage in marijuana smokers that it hides the importance of this simple smoking behavior. *Exhale sooner.* The light-headedness from holding your breath gives an extra rush to the high, but does not increase the psychotropic effects or medical benefits of the cannabis. If you are concerned about even this minor lung irritation, there is a medically-effective alternative—don't smoke it, eat or vaporize it.

STRONGER MARIJUANA

Government statistics from the Mississippi Potency Measuring Project disprove the claim that marijuana is significantly stronger today than it was a decade ago. It's still around 3 or 4 percent THC. However, the proper manicure of a bud before it is consumed improves its potency greatly through the removal of inert plant matter. That part isn't good for you anyway, so you're better off not smoking it—besides, it makes great compost. Most patients with serious illness want strong medicines, especially for allopathic uses. Stronger medicine is better in the case of cannabis, because it means more effective relief with less irritating smoke. This is better for the lungs.

Cannabis is often criticized for having too many chemicals in it. Being a highly evolved organic substance, it contains 421 chemical compounds, sixty of which are medically active. The government declares that it can never approve such a complex substance, while its tax stamp adorns packs of tobacco cigarettes containing over seven hundred chemicals, almost none of which are beneficial. It's hard to argue against such logic.

The synthetic THC pill lacks many of the key beneficial compounds found in ordinary cannabis. This is because the current approval processes of the DEA and FDA are neither sophisticated enough nor designed to handle complex natural medicines like cannabis, which combines a wide range of synergistic compounds into a single therapeutic form. The FDA approval process is designed to handle molecules, not plants. So cannabis chemistry is completely out of their league. The simple solution is to not put cannabis through the "new" drug approval process. Instead, recognize the classical medical literature and recent studies, then grandfather cannabis in as a traditional natural medicine and crop.

ACCIDENT RATES OVERRATED

Public safety is an important concern of society. Concern that cannabis use might lead to injuries is based on the recent, dramatic increase in "emergency room mentions" of marijuana use. The key here is that "mentions of" marijuana is not the same as "caused by" marijuana. In fact, there is little data to support any such connection. The admission process was amended to ask patients if they ever used marijuana, which led to a jump in the reporting. This statistical slight-of-hand created the false impression of dramatic data.

A major source of public safety concern is a Baltimore trauma clinic study, which identified a high proportion of people having active THC in their system when they came into the clinic—almost one out of three. This report has no corresponding studies to replicate it, and the claimed percentage of cannabis use is so disproportionate to the general population as to be suspicious. However, an even more surprising figure is buried in the details of the report. While about half the injuries had been sustained in vehicular accidents, less than 2 percent of the marijuana smokers were driving at the time the accident occurred.[8] In other words, they were the passengers, not the drivers. Cannabis users tend to feel impaired before they actually become impaired, and so are more likely to have a responsible designated driver. That practice should be encouraged.

A major study on driving was undertaken in Holland (to keep American streets free of scientific research), and in 1993 was reported to the sponsoring U.S. Department of Transportation. Researchers identified a "moderate degree of driving impairment which is related to the consumed THC dose. The impairment manifests itself mainly in the ability to maintain a steady lateral position on the road, but its magnitude is not exceptional in comparison with changes produced by many medicinal drugs and alcohol. Drivers under the influence of marijuana retain insight in their performance and will compensate where they can, for example, by slowing down or increasing effort. As a consequence, THC's adverse effects on driving performance appear relatively small."[9]

As far as distraction goes, cannabis does not even begin to compare with common behavioral patterns, such as using a cellular phone while driving. A study showed that people with cellular phones in their cars run a 34 percent higher risk of having accidents than other drivers.[10] Meanwhile, it is feared that the microwaves used in cellular phone communications could damage brain cells or cause other side effects. Evidence assembled by scientists in Australia, the U.S., and Sweden indicates links to diseases such as asthma, Alzheimer's, and cancer.[11] Where are all the double-blind, controlled, clinical research studies the government should have required before it legalized cell phones?

In fact, marijuana is used to distract people from real public safety issues. For example, consider the fifteen people who died and 176 who were injured in a 1987 Amtrak–Conrail train wreck. Almost before the bodies had been recovered from the twisted carnage, a ghoulish group of publicists were trumpeting that the wreck of the *Colonial* had been caused by marijuana. At least two critical mechanical failures were largely responsible for that train wreck, and either one alone could have caused an accident. A warning whistle was disabled, and a signal light was missing from the engine's control panel.[12] All the urine tests in the world will never replace those lives, nor will they solve the mechanical problems that caused that wreck. Three questions arise, then. Why did those who are entrusted with protecting our lives and safety use an anti-marijuana scare campaign to conceal the real causes of this accident, how much evidence in other accidents has been covered up over the years, and who stood to profit from this?

This brings us to the multimillion dollar urine testing industry. Testing for cannabis is a fraud being perpetuated against the working class by government subcontractors. Tests are easy to beat and easy to fail without breaking the law, and when the testing companies make a mistake, they get to charge for a second test to corroborate the first one. They do not measure impairment or ability. They don't give any economic benefit to the firm that pays the bills or the employees forced to submit to this invasion of personal privacy. These tests serve two purposes: to intimidate employees and to make a lot of money for people with little cups and chemistry kits. A government-sponsored study of urinalysis characterized drug testing as "a costly testing procedure [that] . . . says nothing about the individual's work ability, competence or impairment. . . . Drug testing is concluded to be a method for surveillance, not a tool for safety."[13]

Looking for inert cannabinoid metabolites in the hair, urine, and excrement of hardworking Americans—now *there's* something worth eliminating.

HORMONES AND SPERM COUNTS

Men are particularly vulnerable to any perceived threat to their virility, so the Drug War disinformation network aims below the belt. An alarming worldwide drop in human fertility has occurred in the last fifty years. Measured sperm counts have fallen by half. To hear the scare campaigns, you would think marijuana is the greatest birth control device ever invented. In fact, there is a minute, temporary drop in sperm production during the first few months of human male cannabis consumption, but not enough to keep anyone from making babies. A 1974 study found slightly lower mean plasma testosterone in heavy-smoking novices than in a control group, with a "swift return to normal" on abstention from cannabis.[14] High-dosage marijuana intake did not suppress testosterone levels in another study. A group of twenty-seven young men who had smoked cannabis an average of 5.6 years each refrained from smoking for two weeks and were tested. Then they were admitted for a thirty-one–day stay in a locked hospital ward. No cannabis was permitted for six days. Testosterone levels registered in "the upper range of normal adult male levels." Over the next twenty-one days they gradually increased their consumption, some to very high levels, and their hormonal count remained stable.[15]

Once again, hemp has been scapegoated for the real culprit—in this case, probably pesticides. A study by a team of researchers at Copenhagen University compared sperm from fifty-five members of the Danish Association of Organic Farmers, each of whom dedicated at least a fourth of his diet to pesticide-free produce, with samples from 141 airline workers. On average, the farmers produced 43 percent more sperm per milliliter of semen than did the airline workers. This report, in the June 1996 *Lancet*, adds more weight to the growing volume of evidence that man-made chemicals are to blame for the problem. Of course, other factors warrant looking into, such as the fact that the farmers have a cleaner environment and do not eat packaged foods which may contain *phthalates*, chemicals that leach out of packaging materials.[16] If you were the newscaster, which story would you find sexier to report? It certainly is easier to blame marijuana than to learn to pronounce "phthalates!"

MAKING IT UP AS THEY GO ALONG

Many anticannabis crusades are based on the premise that no one will ever read the reports or look at the data that is being misrepresented. Every once in a while they get a surprise.

California legislators claimed in 1991 that the state's "lenient" marijuana laws gave tacit approval for the use of cannabis, and that its decriminalization in 1975 had resulted in a huge increase in marijuana usage. Statistics for the period provided by the Department of Justice, however, revealed that marijuana use had actually decreased during that time period.[17] What had increased was public awareness of the medical benefits of this herb. To counteract the growing reputation of medical marijuana, the California Narcotics Officers Association pronounced in 1996 that "more than 10,000 studies" had found harmful effects from marijuana, citing the University of Mississippi's Research Institute. A Harvard University professor asked the Institute to verify that report. Within a short time, the Institute's research staff flatly denied the CNOA claim. While the research center has a bibliography with more than 12,000 references to marijuana, a spokesperson noted that, "we have never broken down that figure into positive/negative papers." She was "totally in the dark as to where the statement . . . could have originated."

The Drug War is based on the notion that suppressing every use of cannabis, be it medical, industrial, or social, must be maintained without exception to protect children from the evils of drug abuse. Every year since 1980, the laws have gotten harsher, the penalties stiffer, the rhetoric more absurd. Yet surveys of school drug use seem to rise and fall completely of their own accord, regardless of all the posturing. Just as the medical marijuana issue came before voters in California and Arizona in 1996, frightening new reports were released showing a sharp rise in adolescent drug use. They were peddled around by narcotics officers and the prison lobby to campaign against the initiatives. Just weeks before voters took to the polls, new headlines screamed "Teen drug use highest in study's history," and worse "Teenagers' use of drugs may be underestimated."[18] Just one week later, we find this amazing news report: "Just Say No groups mark 10 effective years."[19] Talk about short-term memory loss! If teenage drug abuse is at an all time high, just what effect were these campaigns trying to have on kids? Apparently, the forbidden-fruit effect.

THIS IS YOUR BRAIN ON CHOCOLATE

While research develops new data on cannabinoids and anandamide, recent studies also found that cannabis resin is not the only source of cannabinoids. Three such compounds have now been identified in chocolate.[20] In a statement released by the Neuroscience Institute in San Diego, researcher Daniele Piomelli conjectured that these compounds may "participate in the subjective feelings associated with eating chocolate." Other researchers warn that such conclusions are premature because there is no evidence that chocolate's cannabinoids stay in the body long enough or occur in high enough concentrations to be of any significance. A spokesperson for the Institute of Mental Health estimated that a person would have to ingest the equivalent of 20 percent of their total body weight in chocolate at one sitting to get any psychoactive effect, which means they would get physically sick long before they felt any euphoria.

Cannabis, therefore, clearly remains the best source of natural cannabinoids. Still, this raises important questions about where our bodies get the compounds necessary for our physical and mental health, and how food plays a role in maintaining our chemical balance. And watch out; one day PDFA may target Hershey's, rather than pot, as the stepping-stone drug for kids.

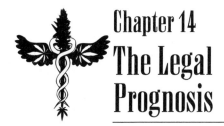

Chapter 14
The Legal Prognosis

A BRIEF HISTORY OF DRUG POLICY

Europeans who settled in America were not lawyers; they were farmers, merchants, and service providers. The fictitious principle that all lands originally belonged to the British king was instituted through the issuance of real estate grants. People readily accepted these titles, since initial rents were low and the papers lent legitimacy to their property claims—as well as providing a handy rationale to drive native peoples off their land. As long as things were going well, there was no urgent reason to expose the pretense, wrote Thomas Jefferson, "but a series of oppressions, begun at a distinguished period and pursued unalterably through every change of ministers, too plainly prove a deliberate and systematic plan of reducing us to slavery."[1] The colonists rose up and asserted their own sovereignty, and wrote a simple Constitution in the clearest English of their day. The federal government existed to defend the land and to protect interstate commerce. Criminal law belonged to the States. Just in case future leaders missed the point, the Bill of Rights was added to clarify the limits of federal jurisdiction: leave the States and the people alone.

It is ironic that this book needs a chapter on legal issues

surrounding cannabis, since drug prohibition is patently unconstitutional, as proved when Prohibition was repealed by the
Twenty-First Amendment. This is why the narcotics police re-
sorted to the smoke screen of a "regulatory" Marihuana Tax Act
of 1937 to suppress cannabis. In a case involving Dr. Timothy
Leary, the U.S. Supreme Court ruled on May 19, 1969, that the
punitive tax is double jeopardy that violates the Fifth
Amendment's ban on self-incrimination. Rather than comply
with the supreme law of the land, however, the drug bureaucracy came up with a system for classifying substances as banned
drugs, Schedule I, then arbitrarily listed hemp in this forbidden
category, while listing hard drugs like cocaine and morphine in
Schedule II, "safe to prescribe." It may no longer be politically
correct to call it prohibition, but to label cannabis "illicit" or
"illegal" is to disguise reality. This violation has been ignored by
the courts under the assertion of a vague overriding interest—a
principle that does not exist in the Constitution—based on crude
Reefer Madness-style propaganda. This has created a de facto Drug
War exception to the Bill of Rights, peppered with selective enforcement, that is equivalent to having federal martial law.

Unfortunately, once Congress created the legal fiction that
banned cannabis, the lesion on the surface of the Constitution
quickly tumored into a bureaucratic cancer that has grown un-
controllably ever since. The United States has the developed
world's highest incarceration rates. Enforcement budgets that
began at a few hundred thousand dollars now surpass $16 bil-
lion per year. A thin hope for cannabis reform policy came during President John F. Kennedy's administration. The United
States had lobbied hard under President Dwight Eisenhower for
the United Nations to adopt the Single Convention Treaty on
Narcotic Drugs, but in 1961 the Kennedy administration decided
not to sign it. Harry Anslinger, the first American "Drug Czar,"
was removed from office, opening up more than a decade of
scientific investigation. The President himself was rumored to
use cannabis for his back pain. His advisory commission on drug

policy made its recommendations in 1963. "This Commission makes a flat distinction between the two drugs [cannabis and heroin] and believes that the unlawful sale or possession of marijuana is a less serious offense."[2] That same year, Kennedy was assassinated, and U.S. drug policy took a turn for the worse, particularly under the leadership of Richard Nixon. In 1968 the United States signed the Single Convention Treaty.

Nixon launched a Drug War against his political opponents. As J. Edgar Hoover said in a 1968 memo to all FBI field offices, "Since the use of marijuana and other narcotics is widespread among members of the New Left, you should be alert to opportunities to have them arrested by local authorities on drug charges."[3] Hoover did not want the FBI to become directly involved in narcotics enforcement, however, because he saw this as the area most likely to corrupt police.[4] Nixon did not share his concern, and announced that, "As I look over the problems in this country, I see one that stands out particularly: The problem of narcotics."[5] Congressional reports state that nearly 15 percent of the soldiers who fought in Vietnam came back to the United States as addicts. While Nixon denounced drugs, the CIA smuggled heroin into the United States inside body bags with dead American servicemen. The agency made billions of dollars between 1967 and 1973 on heroin flown out of Laos in Air America planes.[6] Most of the heroin was refined at a Pepsi-Cola bottling plant in Laos, funded by the U.S. Agency for International Development and promoted in the early '60s by Richard Nixon himself. A House Government Operations subcommittee report made this sublime understatement in 1977: "It was ironic that the CIA should be given the responsibility of narcotics intelligence, particularly since they are supporting the prime movers." Nixon consolidated a number of federal drug agencies into the Drug Enforcement Administration (DEA). He sent D.C. police to disrupt a May 3, 1971, peace rally by arresting as many protesters as possible for pot, and some 8,000 political activists were rounded up and held in Kennedy Stadium until after the protest.[7] A few days later Nixon asserted, "I can see no social or moral justification whatever for legalizing marijuana." When his hand-picked panel of experts came out against criminal penalties on cannabis use, Nixon rejected it. "I will not follow that recommendation." The commission noted the "distinct impression among the youth that some police may use the marihuana laws to arrest people they don't like for other reasons, whether it be their politics, their hair style or their ethnic background."[8]

There was a lull in the Drug War during the Ford and Carter administrations. California and other states decriminalized possession of cannabis. Legalization was generally thought to be close at hand. President Carter asked Congress on August 2, 1977, to end criminal penalties on less than an ounce of cannabis. However, Carter found it politically embarrassing to be portrayed in the media as "soft on crime." He recanted on drug policy and authorized the spraying of Mexican cannabis fields with the deadly herbicide paraquat. Long gas lines and the Iranian hostage crisis sealed his fate in the 1980 election. By that time about half of college freshmen had smoked cannabis, eleven states had decriminalized it, and a few patients in the federal IND program were getting it for free, compliments of Uncle Sam.

Enter Ronald Reagan promising to "get big government off our backs." During his first term Reagan paid little more than lip service to the Drug War, but after his reelection, things got ugly fast. When a little girl at a school auditorium asked her how to avoid drugs, Nancy Reagan spouted, "Why, just say no," and a children's crusade was born. All drugs including cannabis were condensed into one ultimate evil. Media hysteria was whipping Congress and the country into a fury in 1986 when a college basketball player named Len Bias died of a cocaine overdose. It was a personal tragedy that became much more. Bias was the number one draft pick of the Boston Celtics, the beloved home team of Representative Tip O'Neill. On hearing the news, the infuriated House Speaker called his staff together and ordered,

"Give me some goddamn legislation!" The resulting crime bill was a smorgasbord of cruel and unusual punishments, including property seizure, conspiracy law, mandatory minimum sentences for first-time nonviolent offenders, and a nebulous category of "designer drugs" for substances that don't exist. Reefer madness returned with brutal Zero Tolerance enforcement. Normally political opponents, Reagan and O'Neill discovered a common target. Ever since, the two major political parties have tried to outdo each other in a futile, yet expensive, surveillance-and-prison model, plump with their pet projects.

Former CIA director George Bush succeeded Reagan as President. He held out a bag of crack on television and demanded tougher penalties while ignoring evidence that his agency had smuggled tons of cocaine into our country and partially fueled the crack epidemic. When CIA trained Panamanian strongman Manuel Noriega got too cocky about his drug running, Bush made an example of him. The United States invaded the tiny Central American nation, and blasted its governmental compounds back to the stone age with tons of missiles. Noriega was dragged to a Florida prison and locked away, and the drug trafficking went on. But a little-noticed change was underway as the public became better educated about cannabis. A generational shift began to occur, and Bush lost touch with the concerns of the middle-class voter.

While running for office, candidate Bill Clinton admitted that he had opposed the Vietnam war and even tried cannabis while in college, claiming that he "didn't inhale." He spoke out against mandatory minimum sentences for first-time nonviolent offenders. What happened once we elected him? Cannabis arrests went up by 40 percent during his first term of office. He reprimanded Surgeon General Joycelin Elders for voicing support for medical marijuana, and fired her shortly after her guarded comment that we should take a look at "the possibility" of legalizing drugs. He signed a crime bill in 1994 that set the death penalty for growing a tenth of an acre of cannabis—a crop raised by Presidents Washington, Jefferson, Adams, Madison, and thousands of our nation's founders. When voters in Arizona and California voted by large majorities in 1996 to permit medical use of cannabis, the federal drug czar, General Barry McCaffrey, threatened to arrest any doctor that recommended it, and Clinton signed off on the idea. So, once again Americans are enduring a series of oppressions, and the federal government is practicing medicine without a license.

PEREMPTORY LAW

Even lawmakers, lawyers, and judges have a hard time keeping up with all the criminal code changes passed by Congress each year, so the lay person has little chance of sorting out the legal rights and obligations, and often ends up being victimized by the system. Fortunately, the founders of the Republic foresaw that possibility, and prioritized the rule of law. The U.S. Constitution establishes the peremptory chain of legal authority. "This Constitution, and the Laws of the United States which shall be made in Pursuance thereof; and all Treaties made . . . shall be the supreme Law of the Land; and the Judges in every State shall be bound thereby, any Thing in the Constitution or Laws of any State to the Contrary notwithstanding".[9] This means that instead of having to fight over each new layer of laws and regulations, the Constitution determines the real law. When in doubt, go back to the Constitution. Any state or federal law or policy that is in conflict with the Constitution is, in the clarifying language of the Supreme Court's famous *Marbury vs. Madison* decision, "null and void." Since there is no authorization for the government to prohibit drugs, it is clear that the federal ban on cannabis is patently illegal, and every judge is bound by oath of office to disregard or overturn the law. Article 8 of the Constitution allows Congress to regulate interstate commerce, which has been distorted into a claim of "overriding interest" in pursuing the Drug War.

On the other hand, some say that even if the United States wanted to legalize cannabis, it could not do so because of international treaties. Wrong again. The Charter of the United Nations states, "Nothing contained in the present Charter shall authorize the UN to intervene in matters which are essentially within the domestic jurisdiction of any state or shall require the members to submit such matters to settlement."[10] So, unless we're exporting cannabis, compliance is strictly voluntary. Meanwhile, the stated purpose of the United Nations includes, "To reaffirm faith in fundamental human rights . . . [and] To practice tolerance and live together in peace with one another as good neighbors."[11] The right to effective medicine was affirmed in international law in 1948. The Universal Declaration on Human Rights Article 25 provides that "Everyone has the right to a standard of living adequate for the health and well-being of himself and of his family, including food, clothing, housing, medical care and necessary social services."[12] Article 30 reiterates that "Nothing in this Declaration may be interpreted as implying for any State, group or person any right to engage in any activity or to perform any act aimed at the destruction of any of the rights and freedoms set forth herein." As a member of the United Nations, the United States is committed to those principles.

The next vacuous argument is that the World Health Organization and the International Narcotics Control Board have jurisdiction, thanks to a complex web of international drug control agreements designed by self-serving bureaucrats to implement a universal anti-drug policy. When we follow the trail back to the roots of its authority, we come to the Single Convention. The very first sentence of the treaty states that "the medical use of narcotic drugs continues to be indispensable for the relief of pain and suffering and that adequate provisions must be made to ensure the availability of narcotic drugs for such purposes." Article 28 sets three regulations on cannabis: "1) If a Party permits the cultivation of the cannabis plant for the production of cannabis or cannabis resin, it shall apply thereto the system of controls as provided in Article 23 respecting the control of the opium poppy. 2) This Convention shall not apply to the cultivation of the cannabis plant exclusively for industrial purposes (fiber and seed) or horticultural purposes. 3) The Parties shall adopt such measures as may be necessary to prevent the misuse of, and illicit traffic in, the leaves of the cannabis plant."[13] Article 23 requires government supervision of production and distribution of cannabis. So the United States promised to "ensure the availability" of cannabis for medical use, yet refuses to do so based on the hope that none of us will read them. But these agreements indicate that it is a fundamental right for American citizens to use and provide medicinal cannabis, by virtue of the Ninth and Tenth Amendments of the U.S. Constitution.

INDUSTRIAL HEMP BILLS

In light of Article 28 of the Single Convention, described above, drug laws clearly should not apply to industrial hemp, an ecological farm crop with no psychoactive properties. The European Community actually subsidizes farmers for growing seed or fiber hemp. Federal Bureau of Narcotics Director Harry Anslinger assured Congress in 1937 that despite the Marihuana Tax Act farmers "can go ahead and raise hemp just as they have always done it."[14] During the Second World War, the federal government waived prohibition and purchased about a million acres of seed and fiber hemp from American farmers, subsidized the production of processing factories through the War Hemp Industries program, and produced the 1943 USDA film *Hemp for Victory*. At the end of the war, Senator Robert LaFollette said of the Marihuana Tax Act that, "the Senate committee was very much concerned to be certain that in enacting this drastic piece of legislation they weren't putting the Federal Bureau of Narcotics in a position to wipe out this legitimate hemp industry."[15] Nonetheless, it did wipe the industry out after the war and has been eradicating feral hemp ever since.

Senator Joe Galiber of New York submitted two bills reforming cannabis law to the state legislature in 1991. One would have legalized all drugs for adults; the other set a legal age of consent for cannabis use. After discussions with the Business Alliance for Commerce in Hemp (BACH), he added a third bill, to restore the farmers' right to grow industrial hemp as a substitute for timber, cotton, and fossil fuel. The measure got tied up in committee. He tried again in 1992, but to no avail. That year the Library of Congress issued a Report to Congress on hemp, concluding that the federal government was politically opposed to growing it, no matter how beneficial the crop is. In 1994, Hemp Agrotech Corporation in California tried to use the U.S. Department of Agriculture's jurisdiction to plant a privately funded research crop, but state agents went onto federal property to destroy the crop. Also that year, the governor of Kentucky was inspired by the Kentucky Hemp Growers Association and others to appoint a task force to research growing industrial hemp as an alternative to tobacco. In 1995, it issued a statement saying that the government basically would not let them grow it. A University of Kentucky public opinion poll found that about 78 percent of the people were in favor of industrial hemp.

In 1995, Senator Lloyd Casey introduced an industrial hemp bill into Colorado's Judiciary committee with the support of the Colorado Hemp Initiative Project, the Hemp Industries Association, BACH, and local farmers. To almost everyone's surprise, the measure lost in committee by only one vote. This encouraged another bill in 1996, with the support of the Colorado Farm Bureau and the American Farm Bureau. It was approved by the Senate Appropriations Committee, the Agricultural Committee, and a floor vote. Unfortunately, by the time requirements were added for alarms, dogs, guard towers, and eighteen-foot fences, it was so overburdened that it died in the Finance Committee. During the session, Casey was arrested by the Denver sheriff for having a bail of industrial hemp in his senate office.

In the meantime, a Vermont Republican, Representative Fred

Maslack, was moving Act 176 forward through the state Agricultural Committee. He anticipated smooth sailing with the support of his fellow conservatives. By the time the federal government was done making demands, however, and the legislature caving in, the act had gone from allowing farmers to grow hemp to authorizing two years of research without field trials. The victory was almost a setback, because it would have been easier to return next year with a hemp bill that included field trials if it had lost. Now the state is committed to two more years without crops. After releasing the BACH island self-sufficiency development plan, I was contacted by Representative David Tarnas of Hawaii. We discussed different options and he drew up several versions of a 1996 bill to reintroduce industrial hemp as a substitute for sugarcane in the island agricultural economy. When he couldn't get field tests approved for it, Tarnas withdrew the bill. At the eleventh hour, he reintroduced the bill as a research project without test crops. It went through.

Missouri State Senator Jerry Howard also discovered the hemp issue in 1996, and got the state senate to pass a non-binding resolution expressing interest in the crop. It is not a bill, but it commits the senate to seriously consider a bill in the future. The state has a depressed economy, and hemp has strong allies here. Much of the driving force comes from a farmer named Boyd Bansel, whose grandfather introduced rice farming to the area. More hearings are scheduled to put an initiative on the ballot there, perhaps in 1997. Every time state legislators discussed a legal exception for farmers to grow nonpsychoactive industrial hemp, the federal DEA refused to issue horticultural research permits, then threatened to arrest any farmer who tried to grow industrial hemp, forcing the test crops to be canceled.

In Ohio, with the support of the farmers' union and the Ohio Farm Bureau, activists are circulating a citizens petition. The drive has about 25 percent of the 107,000 signatures required to put an initiative on the ballot. And back in Kentucky, actor Woody Harrelson (*Cheers, The People vs. Larry Flynt*) planted four industrial hempseeds into the soil of the Bluegrass State, which was once the nation's largest producer of fiber hemp. Harrelson was arrested on the spot. He is challenging the law against nonpsychoactive seed lines, and faces a year in prison for his political stand.

Drug testing poses a major potential problem for the hemp food industry. In 1996 an employee who had eaten a Seedy Sweetie snack failed a drug test for marijuana. The candy is made by Hungry Bear Hemp Foods using pressed hempseed. Normally it does not contain THC, but apparently a detectable amount of residue from leaves slipped through the cleaning process. Aegis Laboratories found positive readings in one person's urine sixty hours after consuming the candy, and similar cases have arisen in other states. The Department of Transportation issued a policy guide to "never accept an assertion of consumption of a hemp food product as a basis for verifying a marijuana negative. Whatever else it may be, consuming a hemp food product is not a legitimate medical explanation for a prohibited substance or metabolite in an individual's specimen." Rather than recognizing the inherent flaw in its testing system, the DEA is instead considering making hempseed snack bars illegal, since they may occasionally trigger false positives.

Sterilized hempseeds are legally available in the United States, but the sterilization process and shipping costs make it more expensive than other fruits and grains. Fertile seed is strictly controlled, and nearly impossible to get legally.[16] The method used to sterilize the seeds compromises their nutritional value, although to what extent is still subject to debate. Some pest-control processing occurs in the handling of all imported foods, another good reason to allow American farmers to again produce a domestic crop and protect the consumer from such processing. One way to proceed may be a unified response that coordinates the Industrial Hemp Council, the Hemp Industries Association, and political representatives for appropriate responses to each bill that comes up. This will help fight off the legislative encroachment that takes a good bill and turns it into something that really doesn't make the grade in asserting the state's rights and jurisdiction. A coordinated, multistate venture may yet claim the holistic benefits of industrial hemp by establishing reasonable terms of legal compliance.

FEDERAL CANNABIS REGULATION

The United States has provisions for and barriers against medical marijuana on the federal, state, and local levels. The Controlled Substances Act of 1970 devised a comprehensive system of federal drug control laws in the United States. It established five schedules of controlled substances, with Schedule I containing those prohibited from all use, including medical. There is a test for Schedule I drugs, which must meet all three of the following criteria: 1) A high potential for abuse; 2) No currently accepted medical use in treatment in the United States; 3) A lack of accepted safety for use of the drug or substance under medical supervision. Since cannabis is virtually nontoxic and has been clinically demonstrated, historically recognized, and popularly used to help cancer, AIDS, glaucoma, and neurological patients, it clearly fails the second and third tests. In the opinion of the DEA, however, the possibility of cannabis abuse outweighs its own legal obligations. Its arbitrary definition of abuse ("use of any illegal drug equals abuse") is a classic Catch-22 scenario: as long as cannabis is illegal, use equals abuse, ergo cannabis cannot be legalized. The Alliance for Cannabis Therapeutics, among others, fought for nearly two decades in federal court, detailing the case against the ban on medical marijuana, and the DEA's own administrative law judge, Francis Young, handed down his decision in September, 1988. "The evidence in this record clearly shows that cannabis has been accepted as capable of relieving the distress from great numbers of very ill people, and doing so with safety under medical supervision. It would be unreasonable, arbitrary and capricious for the DEA to continue to stand between those sufferers and the benefits of this substance in light of the evidence in this record. . . .The judge recommends that the Administrator transfer cannabis from Schedule I to Schedule II."[17] The renegade DEA refused to comply. The appeals court described that action as "vengeance," noting that the DEA-imposed criteria were "impossible to fulfill and thus must be regarded as arbitrary and capricious. Impossible requirements imposed by an agency are perforce unreasonable."[18] It remanded the decision back to the DEA for explanation, and the next appeals court decided that the question was moot until cannabis was approved by the Food and Drug Administration: another long bureaucratic process that has nothing to do with the tests for Schedule I. And so it goes.

When Congress implemented the Investigational New Drug program in the 1970s to provide cannabis for medicinal use and research, the DEA blocked individuals from enrolling in the program and kept the substance out of the hands of researchers. Thirty-seven state legislatures have voted at various times to recognize the medical value of cannabis, with an average of 87 percent in favor. Archconservative Newt Gingrich was among those who sponsored federal legislation in 1981, 1982, and 1983, to allow medical access to cannabis, asserting that "it was the right thing to do." Even the National Association of Attorneys General found the idea of prosecuting sick and dying people distasteful enough to vote on June 25, 1983, to support legislative efforts "to make marijuana available on a prescription basis to patients undergoing anti-cancer treatment or suffering from glaucoma."[19] But such bills have made little progress. The medical marijuana bill introduced by Representative Barney Frank in 1995, HR 2618, did not make it out of committee, but will be reintroduced.

FIGHTING IN THE COURTS

Faced with the symptoms of debilitating life- and sense-threatening illness, people continue to risk everything to find relief.

With no responsible leadership coming from the administration or Congress, the battles have been left to individual cases before the courts. Most judges are appointed after being prosecutors, not defense attorneys, which gives the prosecution an undue advantage. Given the hard-nosed "tough on drugs" mentality of politics, it is not surprising to find a prevalence of hanging judges over tolerant and informed justices.

Confined to a wheelchair for over twenty years due to an injury, Oklahoma paraplegic Jimmy Montgomery smoked cannabis to stimulate his appetite and help control the severe muscle spasms caused by his injury. Using cannabis allowed him to live in comfort and with relative independence. He kept a low profile regarding his medical use. Based on the testimony of a drug suspect who got a lighter sentence in exchange for testifying against the patient, police got a search warrant and found less than two ounces of cannabis tucked away in a pouch on the back of Jimmy's wheelchair. The judge refused to let him argue medical necessity, but a police expert was allowed to tell the jury that the young man was a drug trafficker, with no evidence of any sales. Based on this unequal testimony, Jimmy was convicted in 1992 of cannabis possession with intent to distribute. To substitute for the cannabis he is no longer allowed to use, the government provided him with opiates, tranquilizers, and muscle relaxants. He was dragged in and out of solitary confinement, handcuffed to a prison bed to restrain his violent spasms, and held without adequate medical treatment for the infections that developed in his lower body. Friends watched his condition deteriorate. After considerable public outcry, Governor Keating released Jimmy to a hospital with electronic monitoring, where he is still deprived of his medicine of choice.

Three elements are usually required to sustain a medical necessity defense in federal court. 1) The defendant did not intentionally bring about the circumstance that precipitated the unlawful act; 2) The defendant could not accomplish the same objectives using a less offensive alternative available to the defendant; and 3) The evil sought to be avoided was more heinous than the unlawful act perpetrated to avoid it.[20] From this legal vantage point, not only must cannabis be beneficial, it must also be the remedy of last resort.

Protecting an operation like a cannabis buyers club requires presenting a general necessity defense. A person is not guilty of a crime who, through necessity, engages in an act that would otherwise be criminal. Necessity is an affirmative defense and is not available in all states. The defendant has the burden of proving by a preponderance of the evidence all of the facts necessary to establish this defense, namely: 1) The act charged was done to prevent a significant and imminent evil, namely, a threat of bodily harm to oneself or another person, or something comparable; 2) There was no reasonable legal alternative to the commission of the act; 3) The harm caused was not disproportionate to the harm avoided; 4) The defendant entertained a good-faith belief that the act was necessary to prevent the greater harm; 5) Such belief was objectively reasonable under all the circumstances; and 6) The defendant did not substantially contribute to the creation of the emergency. These arguments should be advanced to defend medical marijuana providers today.

The concept of proportionality—the penalty should fit the crime—is a bulwark of the justice system. Judges have a lot of discretion in how they make rulings to better serve the interest of justice. For example, Judge Charles Campbell sentenced a Moorpark, California, city official to only one day in jail plus three years probation for political corruption, saying that the experience of being prosecuted constituted sufficient punishment. "Those involved with it every day forget what it can be like for someone to get pulled into the criminal justice system," Campbell said. "They forget what it is like to get arrested, booked into jail . . . to have your life scrutinized in the news. This is probably a nightmare he can't believe he's in."[21] This philosophy should apply to cannabis cases, particularly those suffering the nightmare of chronic illness. In addition, judges and legal scholars, including Chicago's chief federal appeals judge Richard Posner, have come out for legalizing cannabis as a way of reducing crime.[22] But the war on sick and dying people grinds on, day in and day out.

A seldom used but potentially powerful weapon in defense of cannabis patients is the right to sue officials and government agencies, both individually and collectively, for civil rights violations. Under U.S. Code Service 42 § 1983, public officials are not immune from such suits. A patient must establish medical necessity and convince a jury in a civil case that the criminal prosecution violated the fundamental human right to medicine, as established under peremptory treaty agreements. It also applies if the prosecution denied them their freedom of speech, religion, peaceful assembly, or any other Constitutional right.

Under the Religious Freedom Restoration Act of 1993, sacramental use of cannabis is admissible as a First Amendment defense, as long as no commercial activity is associated with the religious use. Medical marijuana is asserted by at least one Christian church to be faith healing, and to deny church members of their faith is a violation of civil rights. Rev. Dennis Shields of the Religion of Jesus Church is using his religious freedom defense in a Hawaii case, based on Genesis 1:29, Ezekiel 34:29, and Revelations 22:1, 2. As an article of faith, medical use does not require scientific proof, being akin to the "laying on of hands" of other churches.

A jury has a right to acquit any defendant, regardless of the laws or the facts of a case, if it believes that doing so furthers the interests of justice. One juror is all it takes to reject the conviction in a cannabis case.

PATIENT BUYERS CLUBS

Many patients grow their own plants, but the garden itself increases their risk, and thereby their anxiety, in using the medicine they find most effective. To minimize their personal risk,

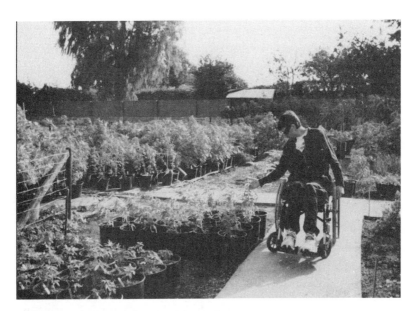

A patient visits a Dutch cannabis garden

patients often group together to form a close-knit community of people they know and trust. They might form a local medical marijuana cooperative or get their herb from a cannabis buyers club that is supplied by commercial growers or importers. Patients and caregivers meet in these self-defined sanctuaries to exchange the herb and share information on their own usage and what they find works best for them. In San Francisco and elsewhere, cases have been monitored by health-care professionals, while clinical research remains blocked at the federal level. As a result, much of the data we have seen in recent years is anecdotal, meaning it comes from the personal experience of an individual rather than a clinical, double-blind study.

Across the country, local patient-operated "Buyers Clubs" dot the nation and are subject to periodic police raids. Offshore from Seattle, Washington, lies rustic Bainbridge Island. One would hardly think that a paralyzed victim of a traffic accident and her husband, living in a small trailer in the woods, would be of any concern to the government. Unless, of course, she uses cannabis to control her pain and improve her overall physical and mental condition. Not only was Joanna McKee doing this, she and her husband, Stich Miller, defiantly provided herb to other patients through the Green Cross Collective, an underground cooperative network of patients and growers. A multijurisdictional drug taskforce, acting on a tip, raided their home in May, 1995. Joanna and Stich were arrested and prosecuted for cultivation and distribution. Several other patients, including people with AIDS, were arrested in the raid. Media reports of sick and crippled people being hauled away in handcuffs for secretly harboring a few square meters of plants embarrassed state officials. Nonetheless, they stubbornly persisted in prosecuting the case and created a national outcry. The charges were eventually dismissed, and Joanna plans to sue the prosecutors who violated their quiet island home. The case helped inspire the state to adopt a bill in 1996 authorizing its university to study the medical utility of cannabis, but the federal government still refuses to release any cannabis for the research.[23]

Seedlings at the San Francisco Cannabis Buyers Club. Courtesy SFCBC.

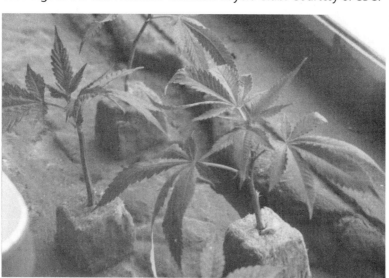

Maria Bruce

The nation's largest buyers club was organized in San Francisco by Dennis Peron in the wake of the AIDS epidemic, after the federal IND program was ended in 1991.[24] Activists put together a City voters' initiative which was passed by voters three-to-one in 1992, expressing support for medical marijuana. Using that vote as a shield, Peron went on to establish his patient-operated club in a five-story building in the heart of the city, with over twelve thousand members and a staff that serviced thousands of clients each week in a casual smoking environment; part clinic, part social organization. To join, patients submit a note from their doctor with a diagnosis of a serious health problem likely to be helped by cannabis. Many people are rejected for insufficient documentation, and bouncers make sure that nobody gets in without a photo ID card. City and county police refused to go after the club, which was prominently featured in many news reports. Activists met there to plan activities. Police operatives under Attorney General Dan Lungren infiltrated the club using forged papers, bought cannabis they claimed was for other patient buyers clubs, and brought minors into the building with them, then secretly videotaped their own illegal conduct. Using this evidence, agents got a warrant and conducted a heavily armed raid of the facility early one Sunday morning, with over one hundred agents, many armed with laser-guided automatic weapons. They humiliated patients and staff, took all the medicine and money, and closed the club to make sure it would serve no more sick and dying people. When the patients turned to the streets, several clergy members of the city opened the doors of their churches to help make up for the shortage. In January 1997 a judge allowed the club to reopen.

Across the bay in Oakland, another model was being developed. This one involved working directly with city officials to seek an element of protection and support. A group of activists, including myself, met with the Public Safety committee to express our concern that a medical emergency exists for certain patients. Discussions led to a hearing on the need for a buyers club, and the staff was instructed to develop a list of options. Ultimately, the city agreed to recognize and protect at least one facility, which now operates as a nonsmoking dispensary and requires a high level of medical documentation for its clients. Since federal law prohibits the *prescription* of cannabis, a diagnosis of serious illness is the core of their evaluation process. The club not only provides cannabis, it helps patients get started in growing their own plants to promote independence, in compliance with the statewide initiative that passed in 1996. Its organizers participate in an advisory committee with members of the city staff and the police departments to implement the letter and spirit of the law.

CALIFORNIA FRONT LINES

California decriminalized cannabis in the 1970s. In 1993 the legislature adopted a joint resolution calling on the federal government to reschedule cannabis as a Schedule II prescription drug. In 1994 and 1995, it passed two bills by large majorities recognizing medical marijuana and exempting doctors and certain patients from state laws forbidding the use of cannabis, both of which were vetoed by the governor. Voters and communities have taken the issue into their own hands by adopting local measures to protect patients and clubs. The bills which Governor Pete Wilson vetoed would have allowed cannabis use only by seriously ill patients suffering from AIDS, cancer, and multiple sclerosis—a very limited category. The California Medical Association and the California Academy of Family Physicians gave their qualified endorsement of the drug for these uses, but the governor disagreed, claiming that the medical use of cannabis would "serve no useful purpose."[25] The only recourse was to turn to the voters.

Momentum had been building in the state for years to develop comprehensive hemp initiative that would legalize industrial hemp and medical marijuana, and set an age of consent for adult social use. In 1992 the effort had gathered 75,000 signatures and in 1994 250,000, all on a shoestring budget. In 1995, I joined activists around the state at a series of meetings and conferences where a large majority agreed to get behind a single-issue, medical reform initiative to express compassion and support for the seriously ill. The general thrust of the measure is that "patients and their primary caregivers who obtain and use marijuana for medical purposes upon the recommendation of a physician are not subject to criminal prosecution or sanction." This includes cultivation of an unspecified number of plants. When it came time to collect the required three-quarters of a million signatures, however, there was no money and the entire steering committee resigned *en masse*. With only a few months to go, we had to create a whole new political structure. Just as things were on the verge of collapse, a group of philanthropists with an interest in the issue formed Californians for Medical Rights. CMR hired a professional campaign manager to oversee the effort. My wife, Mikki, and I were designated to coordinate the community activist aspect of the petition drive, while professional signature gatherers collected the balance. In a monumental effort involving thousands of dedicated people, citizens gathered more than the necessary signatures in just eight weeks in early 1996.

The initiative officially qualified for the ballot and got a number: Proposition 215. Since the polls showed that the public already supported medical use, our strategy was to not make waves. Unfortunately, the prison guards and narcotics police formed an opposing campaign committee. Drug police raided two offices of the campaign, at the San Francisco and Los Angeles Cannabis Buyers Clubs. The official ballot argument against Proposition 215 was signed by Sheriff Brad Gates, asserting in all capital letters that "Proposition 215 is marijuana legalization—not medicine," and the ballot argument signed by the President of the California District Attorneys Association also stated "It is marijuana legalization."[26] Dan Lungren's office stated that "passage would be tantamount to de facto legalization of marijuana."[27] Since making "unfair, deceptive, untrue, or misleading" advertisement is illegal under California law, the assumption must be made that they believe these comments, and would testify to that effect if subpoenaed in a legal case. The federal drug czar made four trips to the state to attack the initiative at taxpayers' expense. The federal Secretary of Health and Human Services, numerous police groups, etc., all similarly ignored the Hatch Act and spared taxpayers no expense in their campaign against the measure, but failed to list these in-kind donations on the campaign report—an elections code violation. Even the Doonesbury comic strip got into the campaign, at which point Lungren unsuccessfully asked newspapers to censor it for criticizing him. Opponents of the initiative argued that allowing doctors to recommend cannabis was tantamount to legalizing marijuana completely, and would open the floodgates of drugs into our schools.

Somehow the voters saw through the special interests and continued to support the measure. On November 5, 1996, California voters passed Proposition 215 by a 12-point margin, 56 to 44 percent. 4,870,822 Californians voted for Proposition 215, as compared with 4,675,552 votes for Bill Clinton and 3,444,493 for Bob Dole. In a less noticed but still significant vote, California voters also overwhelmingly rejected Proposition 205, a jail and prison construction bond bill. With these two decisions, voters sent a clear message to government that they favor reform. But the nonsense did not end when the voters spoke. "The law is so badly crafted, so loosely drafted, that it effectively legalizes the sale of marijuana," Governor Wilson said.[28] Lungren declared the situation "legal and law enforcement anarchy." Proposition 215 proponent Dennis Peron simply replied that, "My opponents said that if people vote for this they vote for the legalization of marijuana, so you can read into it what you want."[29] Even the *Los Angeles Times* opined that the DEA "should review the logic behind its drug schedules. In the meantime, California's only bulwark against marijuana abuse will be the good judgment of its citizens and their physicians."[30] Enabling legislation was drafted, but in the first case of a patient covered by the initiative, Sonoma epilepsy patient Al Martinez, the judge ignored the vote and took the prosecutor's side on every point. The issue may go before the appeals court. Meanwhile, the San Francisco CBC defendants still face trial over the earlier raid.

Lungren said, "We tell people, 'If you don't like a law, go use the process and change it.' Well, despite my best efforts, they changed the law. And we're going to have to live with it."[31] Lungren did add his own spin on the initiative, however, claiming that it would permit use of cannabis "as a last resort," a principle that is not in the law. After a meeting with federal officials, he called on the FDA to step up research, and said that the state's drug police will concentrate on pursuing doctors, growers, and distributors rather than patients. He expressed his concern that the clubs not sell cannabis to persons under the age of 18, to secure parental consent.[32]

RESEARCH OPTIONS

What makes medical marijuana controversial is the fact that it works, and both patients and doctors know it. Otherwise, the federal government would not feel obligated to waste billions of dollars in an absurd effort to deny its medical utility. Few people would argue that prison is better for patients than cannabis, but the mantra of the medical community is that we need more research. The day after Proposition 215 passed, the California Medical Association announced plans to encourage the federal government to conduct controlled studies on the efficacy and safety of cannabis for medical purposes. "The huge voter support of Proposition 215 is really a mandate to the federal government that marijuana must be studied for any medical benefits," said CMA President Jack E. McCleary, M.D. "The CMA will work to encourage research facilities, such as the National Institutes of Health, to conduct studies on the medical value of smoked marijuana to patients." The need for controlled studies is not the only concern of the nation's largest state medical association. The CMA is worried about the threat of federal prosecution of any and all physicians who recommend cannabis. Under the initiative patients need the oral or written recommendation or approval of a physician to possess or cultivate cannabis. It also contains a provision which protects physicians from prosecution under state law; however, physicians may still be subject to serious liability under federal law. "Proposition 215 has absolutely no effect on federal law that makes it a crime to use, distribute, dispense or possess marijuana," Dr. McCleary said. "Proposition 215 may not protect physicians who, in good faith, recommend cannabis for seriously ill patients or compassionate end-of-life care."

Sick and dying people, however, can't wait for political expediency. A medicine grows as a resinous flower on a garden-variety herb, and it is available around the world, and people will continue to use it. Doctors should, therefore, be allowed to oversee it. The AMA's *Code of Medical Ethics* states, "In the making of decisions for the treatment of seriously disabled newborns or of other persons who are severely disabled by injury or illness, the primary consideration should be what is best for the individual patient and not the avoidance of a burden to the family or to society. Quality of life, as defined by the patient's interests and values, is a factor to be considered in determining what is best for the individual."[33]

Without calling for a complete decriminalization of cannabis, a group of scientists on November 15, 1994, called on the federal government to expedite research into the plant's medicinal use for the seriously ill. In a petition to Health and Human Services, the Federation of American Scientists pointed out that whole cannabis is already in clinical use by patients suffering a variety of illnesses, including AIDS and epilepsy. The statement read, "based on much evidence from patients and doctors alike on the superior effectiveness and safety of whole cannabis . . . we hereby petition the Executive Branch and the Congress to facilitate and expedite the research necessary to determine whether this substance should be licensed for medical use by seriously ill persons."[34] Their request was rejected, like all the others. And yet, when the issue reached the ballots, the same government agencies opposed allowing its use on the grounds that there has not been enough research.

Both inpatient studies conducted under well-controlled, experimental conditions and outpatient studies conducted under "real world" conditions are needed to evaluate the safety and efficacy of cannabis. Dr. Donald Abrams, of the University of California at San Francisco, designed a study that combines the two approaches, and has been trying for four years to get permission to conduct clinical research comparing the medical use of smoked cannabis and dronabinol in patients with the AIDS wasting syndrome. Dr. Abrams's proposal was approved by the FDA and all appropriate regulatory authorities. However, the study cannot go forward because NIDA has a monopoly on the supply of cannabis that can legally be used in research and refuses to provide any. NIDA Director Dr. Alan Leshner said he would reconsider the protocol evaluation if it was rewritten as a grant application to the National Institutes of Health (NIH), was reviewed favorably by its evaluation committee, and was awarded government money for the study. This was scant hope, since only 10–15 percent of NIH grants are funded.

Nonetheless, the Multidisciplinary Association for Psychedelic Studies (MAPS) and the Drug Policy Foundation raised $5,000 to pay for staff to prepare the grant application. It proposed two related, sequential studies: first, a randomized, double-blind, placebo-controlled, inpatient evaluation of smoked cannabis at the General Clinical Research Center at San Francisco General Hospital, followed by a randomized, open-label, outpatient study of smoked cannabis versus dronabinol. The inpatient study would provide data on the effects of approximately 4 percent THC-content cannabis on appetite and food intake, as well as safety data on immunological function, HIV viral load, pulmonary function, endocrine function, and neuropsychological function. Based on the results of the inpatient study, Dr. Abrams planned to conduct an outpatient study to develop comparative data on the effects of smoked cannabis versus the licensed, synthetic THC pill. The outpatient study would also provide safety data on immunological function, HIV viral load, pulmonary function, and endocrine function, while treating patients with HIV-associated weight loss over several months.[35]

In late 1996, Dr. Leshner told Dr. Abrams that the NIH had turned him down because the government could not justify the cost of providing cannabis for such a study. The street value of the cannabis needed was only a few hundred dollars—less than the cost of preparing the grant proposal. Even with private funds to provide and evaluate the cannabis, handling it requires DEA authorization, and the FDA can arbitrarily refuse to recognize the study when it is done. So the fox is still in charge of the chickens.

Not to be stymied, Dr. Abrams's research team is submitting a revised protocol which incorporates the NIH critique of its 1996 application to meet the May 1, 1997, NIH cycle deadline. Another research option which has not been pursued in recent years is that of the N=1 trial (pronounced "N of 1"), which is a series of controlled, individual patient studies, rather than studies of large-scale control groups. An effective design criterion was described in the *Journal of the American Medical Association* to produce randomized, double-blind, multiple crossover trial results. "[Single patient trial] costs compare favorably with other conventional services, and clinicians appear to gain confidence and precision from SPTs. When patients or clinicians are uncertain about the value (including the possibility of side effects) of treatment for symptomatic chronic diseases, we believe an SPT can be offered to a patient and will likely yield results that will effect subsequent treatment."[36] The FDA has used these in the past, such as when it approved the use of danazol (a drug used to treat endometriosis) based on a NIH trial involving forty patients, switching between drug and placebo after one month or with an attack. This approach is particularly useful for trials involving chronic, stable conditions or rare diseases, when the treatment offers undetermined benefits but is known to work promptly to provide temporary relief. N=1 trials offer advantages for cannabis research because they are patient-specific in terms of dosage and duration. Outcome measurements, both subjective and objective, are also tailored to the patient. To maintain the double-blind control for a study of THC compared to cannabis, three randomized groups would be given a supply of either A, B, or C. Group A receives 2.5 mg THC for half the test and placebo joints for the second half. Group B receives placebo pills for half and marijuana joints for half. Group C receives placebo pills and placebo joints.[37] Neither researchers nor patients know to which group they belong until the end of the study. Possible objective outcome measures of effectiveness can include patient global assessment, physician global assessment, use of rescue medication, and disease-specific response measurements.

Readers who use marijuana medicinally are urged to participate in the Cannabis Patient Registry (Appendix D). As the possibilities to conduct research evolve, participants may be eligible for inclusion in an N=1 trial.

LEGISLATIVE OPTIONS

The beauty of Proposition 215 is that it does not conflict with federal law because it does not legalize cannabis; it simply creates a medical exception to enforcement. The question of states' rights versus federal domination often comes down to political expediency. For example, when the federal government decided to fight the 1996 anti-affirmative action initiative, Proposition 209, California officials, including Governor Wilson, denounced it as a violation of the Tenth Amendment. However, the governor expressed no such concerns when General McCaffrey threatened to prosecute doctors who recommend cannabis to their patients under Proposition 215 or when the DEA threatened to pull doctors' licenses to prescribe medicine. Dan Lungren went to Washington, D.C., to meet with federal officials to discuss how to get around the new law, and said he was "heartened" by the federal Department of Transportation plan to use urine testing to keep drivers from using medical marijuana.[38] When the U.S. Senate held hearings to discuss the matter, Arizona's Senator Jon Kyl asked the DEA to step up their antidrug efforts in states where voters support medical marijuana.[39] General McCaffrey has repeatedly threatened to use surveillance, entrapment, and secret police to infiltrate and destroy the physicians and clubs that provide cannabis. The intimidation of doctors is extremely problematic because the bill requires a physician's recommendation for cannabis to be used legally. The CMA advised doctors against recommending cannabis, and at least one doctor rescinded his previous recommendation to a patient since the general began his threats.

A special meeting of law enforcement officials, the general, and other opponents of the initiative was convened at taxpayers' expense in Washington, D.C., to thwart the will of the voters. Now there is talk of federalizing the nation's police force by deputizing state and local police to override the will of the voters and defy the Tenth Amendment, an unfunded mandate that borders on treason. And who would pay the salaries of police mercenaries diverted away from enforcing state law to enforce federal law? Taxation without representation is one thing, but being taxed to pay for your own suppression is sadistic.

The Brady Bill provision to control handgun sales by requiring local police to run a background check on buyers was argued before the U.S. Supreme Court in 1996. Justice Anthony Kennedy attacked the plan, asking, "Isn't the point not to have one government interfere with another?" Justice Sandra

O'Connor challenged "the notion that the federal government can just commandeer" state officials to enforce federal law. The federal attorney agreed that the government probably could not require states to administer a federal program without offering them money and a chance to opt out. Those arguments should hold for cannabis, also.

In 1996 in Arizona, voters passed Proposition 200, an even more sweeping bill, by a nearly 2–1 margin. It legalizes prescription and medical use of cannabis and other controlled substances, and replaces prison sentences for nonviolent drug possession with probation. An estimated 1,000 prisoners will be released when it is fully implemented. Proposition 200 was backed by numerous physicians and by prominent Arizona conservatives, including retired Republican Senators Barry Goldwater and Dennis DeConcini, and several former Reagan administration officials. Governor Symington claimed he could veto any proposition that does not receive a majority of the state's total number of registered voters, not only those who voted. "If the governor presumes he has more authority than the people of this state, then he has lived one day too long on the political landscape," House Minority Leader Art Hamilton retorted. He warned that if Symington did attempt to veto the measure, "The first thing I would do in January would be to introduce articles of impeachment."[40] The governor backed down, but the attack moved to the federal level.

A provision allowing cannabis smokers to claim chronic illness or pain as a legal defense was included in the 1996 Ohio state crime bill. When a patient with a Dutch prescription for cannabis was arrested in the state, the new law was invoked in court and discussed in national and international news reports of the case. Charges were dropped due to an illegal search, but after General McCaffrey began threatening to impose federal law, Ohio state legislators claimed that they had no idea what they were voting for. The governor, attorney general, and even the bill's sponsor all denied knowing what was in the law they had adopted. Deputy Attorney General Mark Weaver said, "it's impossible to know what's on every page of every bill passed by the legislature," and promised to have a new bill reversing the law before lawmakers in January, 1997. Ohio voters now wonder what other laws their politicians have unwittingly approved.

Despite these dishonorable political sideshows, the issue is ripe for further development, given the large base of voter support for medical marijuana—about 75 percent, according to a national survey conducted for the American Civil Liberties Union in early 1996. Twenty states now have bills that allow patients to argue medical necessity if charged with cannabis possession. An excellent listing of legal and political options has been compiled by the Marijuana Policy Project foundation into a packet entitled *How Can a State Legislature Enable Patients to Use Medicinal Marijuana Despite Federal Prohibition.*[41] The report is a comprehensive analysis of state medicinal cannabis laws, past and present, as well as recent state legislative proposals. It includes specific suggestions for how activists can approach their officials to enact necessary changes at the state level, and is an excellent starting point for planning such a strategy.

THE FINANCIAL FACTOR

If you judge a plant by the power of its enemies, then cannabis is very important, indeed. How many other garden-variety herbs are listed in national emergency plans, have their own federal eradication program costing taxpayers about $8 billion per year, and generate at least $36 billion in the underground economy each year? Given the broad popular support for medical marijuana and industrial hemp, who, one might wonder, would be opposed to letting sick and dying people use their traditional medicines? Who would forbid farmers to grow a traditional crop that could produce more jobs and clean up the environment? Who benefits from causing so much pain and destruction? Follow the money.

Not only are there multimillion dollar contracts to build and supply our nation's courts, jails, and prisons, now there is domestic prison labor to sweeten the pot for the Drug War profiteers. Federal prisoners in the United States were paid 37½¢ per hour in 1996 to work for the Unicor company; not quite slave labor. That's the same wage paid in 1825 to immigrants working on the Erie Canal. Now there are prisons privately run for profit. In California the prison guard union sleeps snugly with both Governor Wilson, who received almost a million dollars in political donations from the group, and Attorney General Lungren, who's never seen a prison he didn't like. The union was also a major funder of the opposition to Proposition 215.

Alcohol and tobacco companies get big tax write-offs to pay advertising companies to slam their competition, marijuana— as a public service, of course. Pharmaceutical companies sell expensive drugs to replace cannabis, since no one can buy the herb legally. That needlessly drives up medical costs and insurance rates. The drug testing industry has no natural markets, so the federal government passed the Drug Free Workplace bill as a subsidy for this disgusting program, forcing businesses to seize hair and urine samples from innocent, hardworking people without probable cause.

The pork barrel of prohibition is not limited to civilians. The principle of *posse comitatus*, adopted after the Civil War, forbids the military to enforce domestic law, yet the Pentagon has received more than $7 billion for counter-drug operations since the Bush administration overrode that provision in 1989. Rich contracts for exotic equipment are awarded to the same contractors who brought us Vietnam.[42] The military now employs more than 8,000 active duty and reserve personnel as professional drug warriors, and these troops participated in 754 domestic operations in 1995. In a de facto form of martial law, the Defense Department project Joint Task Force Six links the nation's domestic law enforcement forces with soldiers, members of the Air Force, Green Berets, Navy SEALs, and Marine reconnaissance patrols. Along with that, police departments and federal agencies get billions of tax dollars from the government each year to creep around forests, look into backyards, fly overhead in planes and helicopters, and even use satellite surveillance to spy on citizens to see if any hempseed may have sprouted.

If these police happen to catch somebody, the forfeiture laws kick in and allow the agencies to keep a substantial part of any property they seize. The accused don't even have to be found guilty, according to the U.S. Supreme Court.

THE NEXT PHASE

With this book and others, the person who chooses to intelligently self-medicate with cannabis has a chance to make informed decisions. Just as people do not call a doctor to catch a thief, we cannot look to prosecutors, police, prison lobbyists, and criminal lawmakers to dictate appropriate health care for people. Criminal penalties will never successfully suppress cannabis for four key reasons. First, many patients have no choice but to break the law as a matter of medical necessity. Second, cannabis users are recalcitrant offenders because they do not feel like they have committed any crime; in fact, they generally feel proud of their decision to use cannabis and punishment simply makes them lose their respect for government. Third, a policy that is based on obvious lies and conflicts of interest is doomed because the truth cannot be suppressed forever. And fourth, the ecological and economic benefits of industrial hemp are so compelling that the crop will ultimately have to be restored as a matter of planetary survival.

Fully implementing the policy advocated by General McCaffrey after the election entails arresting one out of two cancer doctors, who feel they should in good conscience recommend cannabis to at least one patient, and one out of every three high school seniors, since 38 percent say they smoke cannabis. Whose children are we talking about? Our own. What does that say about his proposal? That it isn't good for our kids.

Parents must not allow the War on Drugs to become a war on young people. We all want to protect our children; the question is how best to do that. Eventually you are going to have to discuss cannabis with your children, and I urge you to be honest and reasonable. Don't live in denial about the real world your children face. If you demand total abstinence from teenagers, you can't talk to them about not driving under the influence, or any of the other gray areas that make up the adult world. Don't underestimate their intelligence. Parents should lead by example to teach their children how to make good choices and control their appetites. That means taking responsibility for the condition of the world you are preparing for them.

Young people will encounter lots of wrong messages about cannabis, many put out by people with good intentions. Marijuana does not kill people, lead to hard drugs, or cause problems in the lives of adults who use it responsibly. Neither is it a toy; it is an important and powerful medicine. It should only be used with parental consent by anyone who is less than eighteen years of age. Certain things require adult judgment, such as voting, driving a car, signing a contract, and drinking alcohol. Cannabis fits into this category, too. There are too many other changes going on in adolescent lives to add to the confusion.

CONCLUSION

Since anyone can develop a health condition that is helped by resinous cannabis, everyone has an interest in creating a safe and affordable distribution system. Political leaders are out of touch with the people on this issue, but they do know how to count votes. We who favor medical marijuana are now an empowered constituency. Each of us can make a personal difference, and together we are a solid majority. The power still belongs to the people, and Americans don't like having their elections stolen.

Now that California and Arizona voters have brought medical cannabis back within the scope of law, we can again hold our public officials accountable for their actions. Civil suits and class actions are appropriate vehicles for this. In January 1997 a group of physicians and patients backed by Americans for Medical Rights filed suit against General McCaffrey and other administration officials for using intimidation to violate their rights regarding cannabis. The nature of the attack on the 1996 elections is just one matter that could eventually lead to grand jury investigations of official misconduct.

When and if patients and doctors are prosecuted in the future, the freedom to self-medicate is likely to be reinforced and expanded by jurors who understand another person's back pain, stress, or religious beliefs. And what will happen when a patient discovers that THC doesn't help, and he needs to grow an acre or two of industrial hemp to get enough herbal matter to extract CBD for his medical need? Sell the stalks for profit, and medical marijuana could well be the stepping stone to industrial hemp!

Many California voters intended Proposition 215 to allow buyers clubs to legally provide affordable cannabis to patients in a safe location. As of this writing, a judicial decision has lifted the injunction against the San Francisco club, allowing it to serve patients again, and numerous new clubs are sprouting across the state. Although dispensaries have their role, it is important that not all clubs become sterile clinics. Cannabis heals the patient's body and mind best in an environment that stimulates health and happiness. Part of what makes cannabis special is that it promotes congeniality and community among its users. Clubs allow patients to share information about their own experiences, as well as socialize in a pleasant, casual atmosphere that lifts their spirits and enhances their recovery.

We can all be inspired by the courageous example of patriots who risk everything to help patients in the darkest hours of prohibition. Just as slavery was the great injustice of nineteenth-century America, so the Drug War is the defining injustice of this century. Dennis Peron, Valerie Corral, Joanne McKee,

Johann Moore, and hundreds of others who openly provide medical marijuana to patients today are the moral descendants of those who once operated the Underground Railroad to rescue African Americans from slavery. Society must learn to recognize the personal dignity and humanity not only of patients, but of all people.

It is no mere coincidence that this book ushers in a new wave of research at the state, federal, and private sectors. Interest in the medical uses of cannabis is expanding at a dizzying pace. Access to hashish, cannabindon (resin extract), tinctures, and other forms of cannabinoids will eventually open still more areas of research. However, the new must always be viewed in the context of what has gone before, so I offer this foundation in hopes that it will trigger further investigations into the therapeutic value of *Cannabis sativa,* true hemp. Perhaps you who read these words will make the next discovery that changes the history of cannabis medicine. The possibilities are wide open, and the future is being written one day at a time.

Hemp for health!

Overall Effects of Resinous Cannabis

The **brain** absorbs THC through unique receptor sites that affect different body systems, triggering a chain of temporary psychological and physiological effects. Initially it has a stimulant effect, followed by relaxation and overall reduction in stress. May cause drowsiness or anxiety. Analgesic effect. Blocks migraine and seizures. Enhances sense of well-being.

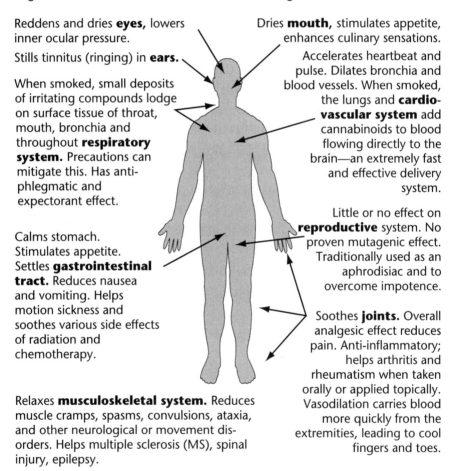

Reddens and dries **eyes,** lowers inner ocular pressure.

Stills tinnitus (ringing) in **ears.**

When smoked, small deposits of irritating compounds lodge on surface tissue of throat, mouth, bronchia and throughout **respiratory system.** Precautions can mitigate this. Has anti-phlegmatic and expectorant effect.

Calms stomach. Stimulates appetite. Settles **gastrointestinal tract.** Reduces nausea and vomiting. Helps motion sickness and soothes various side effects of radiation and chemotherapy.

Relaxes **musculoskeletal system.** Reduces muscle cramps, spasms, convulsions, ataxia, and other neurological or movement dis-orders. Helps multiple sclerosis (MS), spinal injury, epilepsy.

Dries **mouth,** stimulates appetite, enhances culinary sensations.

Accelerates heartbeat and pulse. Dilates bronchia and blood vessels. When smoked, the lungs and **cardio-vascular system** add cannabinoids to blood flowing directly to the brain—an extremely fast and effective delivery system.

Little or no effect on **reproductive** system. No proven mutagenic effect. Traditionally used as an aphrodisiac and to overcome impotence.

Soothes **joints.** Overall analgesic effect reduces pain. Anti-inflammatory; helps arthritis and rheumatism when taken orally or applied topically. Vasodilation carries blood more quickly from the extremities, leading to cool fingers and toes.

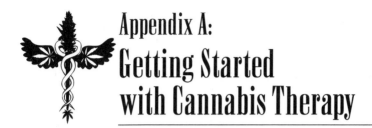

Appendix A:
Getting Started with Cannabis Therapy

Name: Hemp, cannabis, medical marijuana.

Scientific name: *Cannabis sativa* L.

Parts used: Flowering tops, resin, seeds, extracts and cannabinoid analogs.

Dosage: Use only as required to mitigate symptoms. Start very small and build up.

Synergistic effects: Combination with alcohol increases some effects of both drugs. One should not perform any hazardous activity when using cannabis and alcohol simultaneously. Coffee or caffeinated beverages help overcome the drowsiness that sometimes accompanies cannabis use. Calamus is smoked with cannabis in Ayurvedic medicine to add "clarity" and offset some of the effects on the memory, brain, and liver.

Contraindications: Exercise extreme caution if prone to schizophrenic episodes or epileptic seizures, or if suffering from heart conditions. Reduce dosage or discontinue use if excess drowsiness or sense of disorientation interferes with ability to function. Not recommended during pregnancy.

Effective doses: Dosage varies with personal tolerance, herb potency, and the condition being treated. In general, it is better to start with low doses and work your way up as needed. Clinically

Judging the quality of cannabis

Characteristic	Desirable	Undesirable
Aroma	Fresh, sweet, pungent	Earthy, moldy
Moistness	Appears dry but compresses then springs back slightly when pressed gently between fingers; glands are sticky to the touch	1) Appears wet, compacts into a damp mass when lightly pressed; 2) Appears dry, crumbles into an indistinct, powdery mass when pressed lightly
Appearance	1) Plump buds with visible resin glands, glistening with frosty trichomes, red hair; 2) Buds pressed or compacted for shipping, some trichomes visible with a magnifying glass when broken apart	Lots of seed, lots of stem; herb is very leafy or structurally indistinct with no glands visible, even when viewed through a magnifying glass
Freshness	Green, well cured, and smelly	Overly dry, faint or no odor
Manicure	Minimal amount of central stem, hair and calyxes visible, surface coated with resin glands, shade leaves trimmed off	Indistinct mass, leafy, abundant seeds and stems
Cure	Golden color means the herb was cured in sunlight; green or purple buds were cured in darkness	Gray, moldy look
Smoke	White or light blue	Brown, black, sooty

effective oral doses for the relief of nausea start at 5–10 mg THC. Quality marijuana typically ranges from 4 to 10 percent THC. A single cigarette is usually enough for several doses. At 4 percent THC, each one-gram joint contains 40 mg THC, up to half of which may be destroyed by heat or lost as escaping smoke. Not all THC that is inhaled will be absorbed by the lungs. Each dose lasts two to four hours. Eating cannabis releases the active compounds more slowly through the digestive process. This requires more cannabis to be consumed, with its effects lasting two or more times as long as smoked herb, depending on the rate of gastrointestinal absorption. About one-half to one gram of cannabis per oral dose is standard, but this varies widely according to herbal potency. No standard dose has been established for CBD or other non-marijuana cannabis compounds.

Toxicity: Occasionally, people may get too resinated for their personal comfort, but their bodies will still function fairly normally. Simply put, cannabis is nontoxic. The low toxicity of THC is evident in its widespread use by millions of people without a single death ever by overdose, and very few reports of anything even approaching lethal overdose. About one gram of THC per 1,000 grams of body weight is projected as being its potential LD-50, meaning a lethal dose for 50 percent of any group of organisms that consume this amount. This means that an average-sized human being would have to consume 50–100 grams of pure THC in just a few hours to reach that level: anywhere from one and three-quarters to four U.S. ounces of the isolated compound. Since high-potency cannabis is only about 10 percent THC, a person would have to eat a minimum of one or two pounds of top-grade marijuana within a couple of hours to have even half a chance of dying from it. Accounting for heat and smoke loss, one would have to smoke at least twice that much. In short, a potentially lethal dose of THC is several thousand times more than its effective medical dose. For alcohol, the difference is only about twenty times, and other common nonprescription drugs, such as aspirin, have similarly narrow margins of safety.[1] This is why cannabis has been determined to be "one of the safest therapeutically active substances known to man."[2]

Additional warnings: 1) Smoke causes minor bronchial irritation that can lead to bronchitis in extreme cases. 2) Extra caution is recommended for novice users. 3) Avoid driving and operating heavy equipment. 4) Nonaddictive, but may be habit forming. 5) Current drug policy may result in arrest of patient and practitioner, criminal prosecution, asset seizure, separation from family, and longterm imprisonment.

HEALTH AND SAFETY TIPS
FOR CANNABIS CONSUMERS

The herb should be in good condition. Remove all the seeds and as much stem as is practical. There are no medicinal compounds in either of these. Separate out the bigger leaves for cooking, and manicure the buds to your preferred condition. Store the herb in a sealed jar and keep cool and dark, if possible, to maximize shelf life. The buds should be cured and dried to a moisture content of 10 to 15 percent. Never store damp cannabis, because it can ferment, mold, or decompose. Herb should be kept dry enough to prevent fermentation and avoid the development of fungus. The most likely secondary health risk identified with smoking cannabis is that of aspergillus mold exposed to people with compromised immune systems. Suspect cannabis should be heated in an oven for three minutes or more at a temperature of 220°F (104°C). Alternatively, it can be microwaved at high power for at least a minute, as a precaution. This will kill the bacteria without affecting potency. It will also overdry the herb, which will make it burn hotter as a result, so don't overdo it.

Eating resinous cannabis does not irritate the lungs like smoking does, but it has many of the same therapeutic benefits. The overall effect can be very different, sometimes making the patient feel more tired than smoking does. There are important differences between the two methods, in terms of gauging dosage, speed of onset of the benefits, and duration of the effects. During digestion, the liver hydroxylates THC, increasing the potency. So, when eating cannabis it's possible to use lesser quality herb and higher quality cannabis leaf to gain added value from the garden. This also works for consuming CBD, which is more prevalent in less potent cannabis. However, because it's easy for the patient to accidentally eat too much cannabis, always start with a smaller dose than you think, and wait at least two hours before taking in another small amount, if needed.

Don't touch your lips to a shared joint or pipe. This is a definite way to transfer germs between individuals. Whenever possible, don't share smoking utensils, particularly not with anyone whom you know is contagious. Always allow the glue on a joint to dry completely so that bacteria will not be transmitted. Each patient should have their own joint or smoking device, if possible. If you find yourself in a social setting where people pass a joint around in a group, hold it so that your lips only touch your own fingers, not directly on the paper which has been in contact with anyone else's mouth. Also use your fingers like this to smoke a shared pipe. A relatively safe way to share a pipe is to use a chimney-like pipe called a chillum, which smokers hold upright in their cupped hands. In India, Sadhus also wrap a piece of cloth around the base of the chillum to filter out particulate matter. A patient can hold a joint like a chillum as it is smoked, also, which adds a cosmopolitan atmosphere and makes the experience safer for everyone.

Don't get burned. The small remains of a burning joint, called a roach, can be relatively hazardous, particularly if the joint has been rolled too loosely. Many patients have had the unpleasant experience of burning their fingers while trying to take that last precious puff on a roach. Even worse is to inhale the burning embers of cannabis itself, which can occur from either a joint that is breaking apart or a pipe that is smoked without a screen. These painful burns can last for days. There

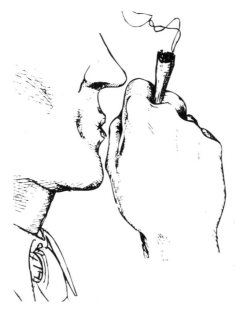

1. Using a one-
handed chillum
technique.

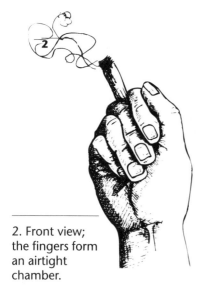

2. Front view;
the fingers form
an airtight
chamber.

3. Inhale through the
opening between the
thumb and index
finger.

are several ways to avoid this problem. One is to use a paper card-stock filter, like they do in Europe—often a piece torn from a matchbook, cigarette paper packaging, or a business card. Use only clean, nontoxic materials to make a filter. This does a double service. It ensures that there is something left to hold onto all the way through the smoking process, which protects your fingers, and it creates a barrier against any stray cinders that might otherwise have been inhaled. If a piece of punctured aluminum foil is used as a pipe screen, heat it up before using it so that any oxidation of the metal occurs before you inhale through it.

Take in enough air with the smoke. It can be difficult to keep moist hemp flowers or the concentrated resins burning at a steady rate, especially when rolled into a joint. Once the smoking technique has been mastered, many people learn to savor and enjoy the sweet flavor of gourmet cannabis smoke. With experience, the patient learns that by taking in some fresh air from the side of the mouth, they can moderate the density of the smoke they inhale. Many smoking pipes now come with a small air hole that can be blocked with the finger or opened to regulate the mixture of smoke to outside air. This ventilating hole is called a carburetor, like in a car engine. It allows the smoker to concentrate the smoke into a chamber, exhale and then take in all that smoke at once, and finally let in fresh air at the end of the inhalation to clear out the pipe stem and chamber.

Don't hold smoke in your lungs very long. It doesn't make much difference in terms of medicinal intake. The most active interchange of medical compounds occurs almost immediately as the smoke is taken into the lungs. The bronchodilation effect relaxes the muscles and expands the bronchial tubes within the lung, which transfers cannabinoids into the bloodstream very efficiently. This process occurs within a matter of seconds, after which the ratio of potentially destructive compounds increases. In other words, holding the smoke longer increases the health risks more than it increases the THC intake.

Don't mix cannabis with tobacco. This may seem obvious in

America, but it is common practice in Europe. Tobacco is treated with chemicals that help the cannabis burn more smoothly, but I highly discourage mixing the two. Tobacco smoke is deadly and does severe damage throughout the lungs. Furthermore, tobacco blocks several health benefits of cannabis. For example, cannabis is a vasodilator, and tobacco is a vasoconstrictor. Cannabis is a bronchodilator, tobacco is a bronchoconstrictor. Cannabis stimulates appetite, tobacco suppresses it. Cannabis is an overall relaxant, and tobacco is an overall stimulant. The difference is like day and night.

Consider using a "bong" or water pipe. Many smokers feel that the bong ensures maximum efficiency in the smoking process. These smoking systems cool the smoke and filter out any ash that may be sucked through the bowl of the pipe. This allows the patient to inhale a larger dose of smoke. Small-sized bowls that hold a single hit, or inhalation of smoke, reduce smoke loss into the air and economize the use of cannabis. Although there is also some loss of active compounds into the water, it is not a critical amount. Do not, however, filter cannabis smoke through wine or any other alcoholic beverage, because the oil-based active compounds will dissolve in the alcohol, resulting in a higher loss of medical benefits. Resist the temptation to drink the bong water. Not only does it taste horrible, but most of the stuff that it has filtered out is not anything you want to consume, anyway.

Use solar energy to light up. Sulfur from matches, carbon monoxide from butane lighters, soot from candles—who needs them? On a sunny day, a patient can use a good magnifying glass to focus sunlight directly onto the cannabis in their pipe or cigarette and ignite the herb with none of these harmful byproducts. Don't stare at the point of combustion too long, though; it can cause a temporary sun spot in your vision.

Vaporize the resin. The most active cannabis compounds are rare in the vegetative matter but concentrated in the resin glands. These glands are actually a thick, oily compound that heats up, liquefies, boils, and turns into vapor without combusting. This occurs at a lower temperature than that at which the plant's lignocellulose starts to burn and give off smoke. Therefore, by maintaining the correct temperature range, it is possible to consume most of the active compounds without ever igniting the herb, which oxidizes the carbons and forms ash and cinder. This occurs in the 300° to 400°F temperature range, but varies according to the altitude, diameter of the bowl, distance between the heat source and the herb, and so on. The process should be visually monitored so that only a transparent vapor is rising from the cannabis, not thick smoke. Paintstripping heat guns can be adjusted to achieve the optimum temperature. Several vaporizers are now on the specialty market, which collect the fumes in a chamber to be inhaled once there is enough vapor for a measured hit.

This is by far the cleanest way to inhale the fumes, producing a sweet but subtle aroma and flavor. Because vaporization is so clean, patients may not realize that they've taken in as much as they have, so go easy with it. After a few tries, you'll come to recognize the burnt taste that means the resin has been vaporized and the flower itself is beginning to roast. Resist the temptation to continue beyond this point, or it's back to smoking. When the resin is gone, the bud's interior begins to look light brown, its structure becomes weak and powdery dry, and it begins to crumble. Even though the bud may still look good, the leftover plant matter should not be smoked. It is not yet clear how this affects the proportion of cannabinoids being consumed, so some people use the leftovers for baking. I recommend composting it.

Appendix B: Cannabis Therapy Reference Table

Condition	Method of application	Therapeutic effect
Abrasion, superficial skin injuries	Resinous herb applied topically; extracts; topical decoctions of roots	Antibiotic, antiacterial
AIDS	1) Resinous herb smoked or eaten; tinctures used; 2) Hempseed or oils eaten	1) Relieves side effects of AZT and chemotherapy; helps control pain, nausea, vomiting, syndrome; insomnia, depression, loss of appetite, wasting 2) EFAs in seed oil bolster immune system
Anorexia	Resinous herb smoked or eaten	Stimulates appetite, increases enjoyment of food, increases intake of liquids (due to dry mouth)
Anxiety	CBD extract	Anxiolitic
Appetite	Resinous herb smoked or eaten	Stimulates appetite, increases enjoyment of food, increases intake of liquids (due to dry mouth). May also reduce appetite or distract people from hunger.
Arthritis	Resinous herb smoked or applied topically	Pain relief, anti-inflammatory
Asthma	Resinous herb smoked	Bronchodilation, improved breathing, anti-inflammatory
Ataxia	Resinous herb and CBD extract	Relaxes muscles, increases smoothness of movement

Bloating, holding water	Resinous herb smoked or eaten, tincture	Diuretic, increases urine flow
Bronchoconstriction	Resinous herb smoked	Dilates bronchia
Burns	Topically applied decoction of root	Soothes pain, speeds healing
Cancer	1) Resinous herb smoked or eaten	1) Relieves side effects of radiation and chemo-therapy, such as loss of appetite, wasting syndrome, nausea, and vomiting; Helps control pain, insomnia, and depression
	2) THC applied to tumor	2) May reduce size of tumor
Childbirth	1) Seed oil applied	1) Soothes skin, lubricates orifice, reduces stretch marks
	2) Hempseed eaten	2) Keeps mother healthy; later helps wean baby from nursing
Chronic fatigue syndrome (CFS)	Resinous herb smoked in large doses along with exercise and posture control	Energizes, motivates individual, allows introspection
Concentration*	Resinous herb smoked or eaten	Provides focus, reduces fatigue
Congestion	Resinous herb smoked	Expectorant—coughing causes phlegm to break up to be spat out. Dries up mucus membranes
Constipation	Hempseed eaten or taken boiled in water	Lubricates intestines, softens stools
Cough*	Tincture	Reduces throat tickle
Cramps	Resinous herb smoked or eaten	Relaxes muscles, relieves cramping

* Extra caution urged, because under certain conditions cannabis can trigger episodes, as well as treat them.

Condition	Method of application	Therapeutic effect
Creativity	Resinous herb smoked or eaten	Encourages nonlinear thinking and tangential or allegorical connections to be made
Depression	Resinous herb smoked or eaten	Raises spirits and stabilizes mood, helps motivate the patient to act
Diarrhea	Hempseed eaten or taken boiled in water	Soothes intestines, solidifies stools, helps reduce loss of liquids and nutrients
Digestive disorders	1) Resinous herb smoked or eaten 2) Hempseed eaten	1) Stimulates appetite, increases enjoyment of food, increases intake of liquids (due to dry mouth) 2) Provides nutrition, lubricates bowels, supplies edestin and EFAs
Drug dependence	Resinous herb smoked or eaten	Used for drug substitution and to ease with drawal symptoms
Dystonia	CBD extract	Relaxes muscles, eases spasms
Ears	1) Resinous herb smoked or eaten 2) extracted juices poured in ear 3) seed oil ear drops	1) Reduces ringing in ears 2) Disinfects ear, reduces pain 3) Loosens earwax for removal
Epilepsy*	Resinous herb or CBD extract	Anticonvulsant; prevents onset of seizures, reduces severity of seizures, speeds up recovery
Eyes	Resinous herb smoked or eaten, eye drops	Treats glaucoma, eye fatigue, ocular headache

* Extra caution urged, because under certain conditions cannabis can trigger episodes, as well as treat them.

Condition	Preparation	Effect
Fatigue	Resinous herb smoked or taken in homeopathic tincture along with exercise regimen	Reduces tedium, fatigue, and boredom with tasks
Fever	Resinous herb smoked or eaten, cool herbal bath	Lowers body temperature, promotes rest
Glaucoma	Resinous herb smoked or eaten; eye drops	Dries eyes, lowers intraocular fluid pressure
Hair	Hempseed oil-based shampoos, conditioners	Moistens, conditions, softens, cleans, stimulates, adds shine, cleans follicles
Hallucinations*	Resinous herb smoked or eaten, tincture	Reduces occurrence and impact of hallucinations in psychosis and psychedelic states of mind (LSD)
Herpes	Topically applied herbal poultice or THC extract	Antibiotic, pain relief, shortens duration of attack
Huntington's disease	CBD extract	Antispasmodic
Hygiene	1)Hempseed oil products	1)Soaps, cleaning agents
	2) Resinous herb extract	2) Disinfectants
Infection	Resinous herb or extracts applied topically	Antibiotic
Inflammation	Resinous herb smoked, eaten, or applied topically	Anti-inflammatory, pain relief
Insomnia	Resinous herb or CBD extract	Increases both deep sleep and REM sleep

* Extra caution urged, because under certain conditions cannabis can trigger episodes, as well as treat them.

Condition	Method of application	Therapeutic effect
Lips	Hempseed oil balm	Moisturizes and smoothes lips
Manic depression	Resinous herb smoked or eaten	Moderates mood cycle
Memory*	Resinous herb smoked or eaten, tinctures	Helps in cases of senility to retain long-term memory. Accesses sensory-linked information learned while under the influence. Caution: may distract short-term memory.
Menopause	Resinous herb smoked or eaten, tinctures	Eases headache, mood shifts
Migraine	Resinous herb smoked or eaten; tinctures	Eases pain, acts as prophylactic to prevent migraine attacks
Miscarriage	Resinous herb smoked or eaten	Reduces cramps and spasms, relaxes muscles, speeds up the process, eases pain
Multiple Sclerosis (MS)	Resinous herb or CBD extract, tinctures	Helps control spasticity, ataxia, eases pain and cramping
Neuralgia	Resinous herb smoked or eaten	Analgesic
Nursing mothers	Hempseed eaten or taken boiled in water or milk	Stimulates lactation, increases available GLA in mother's milk
Nutritional deficiencies	Hempseed, seed oil	Provides EFAs and essential protein
Overachiever complex	Resinous herb smoked or eaten	Allows individual to relax, usually reserved for evenings or weekends

* Extra caution urged, because under certain conditions cannabis can trigger episodes, as well as treat them.

Condition	Form	Effects
Pain	Resinous herb smoked or eaten, THC or CBD extracts	Sedative, analgesic, not full anesthetic, distraction from pain
Phantom limb	Resinous herb smoked or eaten	Reduces imaginary sensations, such as itching or discomfort
Phlegm	Resinous herb smoked	Expectorant
Premenstrual Syndrome (PMS)	Resinous herb smoked or eaten	Eases cramping, depression, moderates mood swings
Psoriasis	Hempseed oil, EFA, lotion	Moisturizes skin, soothes itching
Psychosis*	Resinous herb or CBD extract	Eases depression, moderates mood swings
Rheumatism	Herb or extracts applied topically	Pain relief, anti-inflammatory
Rhinorhea (runny nose)	Resinous herb, smoke inhaled through nose	Dries mucus membranes
Scalp	Resinous seed oil-based shampoos	Moistens, conditions, stimulates, replaces EFAs on epidermal layer of cells, clears hair follicles to facilitate new growth
Sex drive	Resinous herb smoked or eaten	stimulates blood flow to genitalia, heightens overall sensuality; may distract to other interests
Sickle cell anemia	Resinous herb smoked or eaten; hempseed oil eaten or used as massage oil	Pain relief, elevates mood, eases movement, boosts immune system
Skin dryness, itching, chapping, eczema	Hempseed oil, lotions, creams, salves, balms	Soothes, moisturizes, conditions, replaces EFAs on epidermal layer of cells

* Extra caution urged, because under certain conditions cannabis can trigger episodes, as well as treat them.

Condition	Method of application	Therapeutic effect
Sleep	Resinous herb or CBD extract	Induces sleep, encourages deep sleep, and increases REM sleep
Spasticity	Resinous herb or CBD extract	Prevents or reduces muscle spasms and cramps
Spinal injury	Resinous herb smoked or eaten	Helps control pain, spasticity, and depression
Stress	Resinous herb smoked or eaten	Reduces tension and anger
Terminal illness	Resinous herb smoked or eaten, tinctures	Instills sense of acceptance and well-being, reduces pain, allows patient to face death with dignity
Tinnitus	Resinous herb smoked or eaten, homeopathic tincture	Reduces ringing in ears
Tourette's syndrome	CBD extract	Helps control physical twitches and verbal outbursts
Tuberculosis	Resinous herb or CBD extract, hempseed eaten	Helps control dietary disorders and allows patient to eat more normally
Urinary tract problems	Resinous herb smoked or eaten, tinctures	Mild diuretic, helps with cystitis
Vomiting	Resinous herb smoked	Antiemetic
Wasting syndrome, phthisis	Resinous herb smoked or eaten; seeds eaten or taken boiled in water	Stimulates appetite, increases enjoyment of food, increases intake of liquids (due to dry mouth)
Withdrawal	Resinous herb smoked or eaten, tinctures	Eases pain, distracts mind

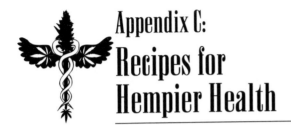

Appendix C:
Recipes for
Hempier Health

HEMPSEED RECIPES

Mellow Vinaigrette

This salad dressing highlights the naturally nutty flavor of hempseed oil. It is ideal for green salads, pasta salads, or other cold dishes. Do not cook with hempseed oil, as the healthful EFAs are broken down by heat. Mix $^2/_3$ c. hempseed oil, 1 tbs. balsamic vinegar, 1 tbs. lime juice, 1 tbs. orange juice, a pinch of cumin, and a pinch of salt together in a glass jar. Store in the refrigerator for up to 2 weeks.

The following recipes are from the *Hemp Seed Cookbook,* by Carol Miller and Don Wirtshafter. It can be ordered from The Ohio Hempery by calling 1-800-BUY-HEMP.

Hempseed Meal: the basis of hemp cooking

First wash the seeds several times. Select only the seeds that float. Immediately dry roast in a heavy skillet on top of the stove, or at a low temperature (250–300°F) in the oven. Roasting will take 5 to 10 minutes. You will know they are done when they stop popping and begin to smell like roasted nuts. Avoid

French roasting. Cool the seeds and grind. Any grain grinder, nut grinder, or coffee mill will work. To reduce the coarse texture of the hulls, you may want to flash blend the toasted seeds briefly, then sift out the fragments. For a buttery texture, you may want to grind twice.

Hempseed and Walnut Loaf

In 2 tbs. olive oil, saute 1 c. chopped herbs (oregano, cilantro, parsley, basil—any or all), 1 lb. chopped onions, 1 c. chopped mushrooms, 1 c. chopped carrots, 1 c. chopped cabbage (or chard, zucchini, or other seasonal vegetables), $1/2$ c. chopped celery, and 4 crushed garlic cloves. Add and mix together: 1 c. hempseed meal, 3 c. walnuts, 1 c. cooked rice (part wild rice is nice), 3 tbs. tamari or soy sauce, 1 lb. mashed tofu, $1/2$ c. nutritional yeast. Press into 9" x 13" baking dish. Sprinkle with a thick layer of nutritional yeast. Bake for 35 minutes at 325°F, or at 300°F in a glass baking dish. Cut into squares. Smother with mushroom gravy. Optional additions: 1 c. cheddar cheese, shredded; 4–6 eggs, beaten. Serves 12–16.

Hempseed Chocolate-Almond Torte

Whip $3/4$ c. butter or margarine. Beat in 6 egg yolks, one at a time. Mix in 1 c. melted chocolate chips, $1^3/4$ c. ground almonds (about 1 lb.), $1/2$–$3/4$ c. hempseed meal. Beat until stiff: 6 egg whites. Fold in. Put into two 8- or 9-inch round cake pans. Bake for 10 minutes at 375°F. Lower heat to 325°F and bake for another 20 minutes. Cool before frosting. Serves 12–16.

Porridge (Gruel)

In a small pan, combine: 1 c. toasted, ground hempseed and 2 c. water, or more if you prefer. Heat to boiling, then turn heat down and cook 5–10 minutes. Remove from heat and let stand until it is the consistency you want. Sweeten with maple syrup or honey and serve with milk.

The following recipes are from Roger Christie's *Gourmet Hempseed Cookbook.*

Hemp Smoothie

Place $^1/_2$ c. roasted hempseeds, 2 ripe (or frozen) bananas, $^1/_2$ c. plain or vanilla yogurt, and fresh or frozen fruit of your choice in a blender with 3 inches of water or fruit juice. Blend thoroughly for a delicious, nutritious protein drink. What a way to start the day!

Hemp 'N Honey Spread

In a serving bowl, mix 1 c. roasted ground hempseed with enough fertile hempseed oil (or olive oil) to moisten the mixture; add honey to taste. Spread on bread or crackers or use as dip.

Spirulina Hemp Date Nut Balls

Mix 2 c. dates, pitted and mashed, $^1/_2$ c. roasted ground hempseed, $^1/_2$ c. chopped macadamia nuts, $^1/_4$ c. powdered spirulina, and 2 tbs. honey. Form into balls. Roll in flaked coconut for a sweet and healthy treat.

The following recipes are from the sixteenth-century *Pen T'sao Kang Mu,* translated from the Chinese by Norman Goundry. They can be found in Kenneth Jones's book *Nutritional and Medicinal Guide to Hemp Seed.*

Beneficial Chi

Boil 2 l hemp seed with 1 l soybeans. Drain and fry slowly, stirring to make a dried powder. Roll the powder in honey as a binder and make into pills. Take twice a day to assuage hunger for long periods.

Black Gold Powder

Thoroughly clean hemp seeds, roast, and crush into a fine powder. Apply topically to treat abscesses, boils, pimples, and swellings.

Nutritional Supplement

Place 604 g of ground hempseed in water, soak, and strain to obtain a juice. Add two-tenths of a liter polished, round grain, non-glutinous rice and boil to a thin porridge. Add to the porridge several salted, fermented soya beans; the bottoms of Chinese green onions; and a condiment of roast prickly ash and salt. Eat when the stomach is empty for relief from various forms of paralysis (palsy), rheumatism, and numbness, or to ease obstructed bowel movements.

Hair and Cough Formula

Boil hemp seeds until they become black. Remove the seeds and extract the oil by crushing the seeds. The remaining liquid can be used as a drink to soothe the throat and stop coughing. The extracted oil, *ma you,* is applied to the scalp to clean the pores and feed the hair roots. Used to cure excessive hair loss and stimulate overall hair growth.

RESINOUS CANNABIS CONCOCTIONS
Bhang Milkshake

The classic Hindu cannabis beverage, in which cannabinoids are suspended in the fatty content of milk, making digestion faster and easier. Take 220 grains cannabis; 120 gr. each of poppy seed, pepper, almonds, and cucumber seed; 40 gr. ginger; 10 gr. each caraway seed, cloves, cardamom, cinnamon, and nutmeg; 60 gr. rosebuds; 4 oz. sugar; and 20 oz. milk. Boil together and cool.

Cannabis Butter (Ghee)

1 oz. finely chopped cannabis flowers, 2 qt. water, 1 lb. butter. Combine ingredients in a large pot, bring almost to a boil, and simmer at very low heat for 24 hours. Remove from heat, add honey, and strain through cheesecloth. Discard solids. Allow butter to rise to the top, and skim off into a separate dish. Discard the water. Butter is ready to be wrapped and stored. Cool

and use. It can be frozen. Test for potency before adding to any recipe. Reduce the butter or shortening called for in the regular recipe by an equivalent amount of cannabis butter.

Curing Cannabis Flowers

Uproot plant or cut low on stem, and hang upside down by the base to let the sap flow into the flowers. Remove and separate large shade leaves for compost or making shake. Hang in sunlight for a golden color. Hang in dark, warm, and well-ventilated place to retain green color. Can also be dried lying down, as long as it is turned occasionally. If using an ionizer in the drying room to avoid odors, be aware that it will reduce the flavor and fragrance of the cured herb. When the moisture level is down to about 12.5 percent, it springs back more quickly when squeezed. The ideal moisture content for use or storage is 10 percent. Cannabis is best when it is fresh. Since oxidation reduces the potency, delay the final manicure until shortly before consuming the herb. Store in a glass container in a dark, cold environment to retain maximum potency, taste, and aroma.

Fresh Cannabis Juice

Prune off some fresh cannabis flowers. Lightly rinse them under cold water and cut the flowers into pieces of suitable size to fit into a juice extractor. Run at a speed to liquefy. Remove lignocellulosic plant matter and compost it.

A few drops of extracted juice can be dabbed onto the skin as a topical ointment, placed under the tongue for absorption, or added to a cup of tea or fresh water and drunk. Fresh juices should be used as soon as possible after preparation; however, if you place the liquid in a small glass container, cork it tightly, and refrigerate it or keep it in a cool, dark place, it will last for several days without appreciable loss of effect.

Hashish

Take cured cannabis flowers and carefully sift off the resin. Gather together the resin glands (trichomes) and roll them into a ball or compact into a gummy, sticky mass. Try to avoid having it come into contact with external oils, such as from your hands.

Hash Brownies

Hashish and chocolate are a fine combination, since they both contain cannabinoids. In Spain, Brazil, and Portugal, "chocolate" is slang for hashish. Many people feel that adding resin to brownies is better than using herbal cannabis because it is smoother in texture and has a distinctive flavor.

Pulverize 5 g of hashish. In a separate pan over hot water, melt 2 oz. unsweetened chocolate and $^1/_3$ c. butter. Add the hashish. Beat in 1 cup sugar and 2 eggs. Sift together and stir into the mixture $^3/_4$ c. cake flour, $^1/_2$ tsp. baking powder and $^1/_2$ tsp. salt. Mix in $^1/_2$ c. roasted hempseed. Pour into a greased 8-inch square pan. Bake for 30 minutes at 350°F. Nibble with caution.

Herbal Pack or Plaster

Soak large cannabis leaves in strong isopropyl alcohol for two weeks. Remove singly and wrap around stiff, aching joints. Dried flowers or leaves soaked in alcohol for the same period can be mashed into a paste and applied to affected areas and under wrappings.

Herbal tinctures

Loosely fill a glass bottle or jar with cannabis flowers. If using fresh plant matter, cut it up with a scissors; if dried, crumble it up. Add pure spirits—use drinking alcohol (ethanol), not rubbing alcohol (isopropyl) or denatured alcohol. A liquor like vodka or whisky with a high proof rating will do nicely. The flavor of the liquor will affect the flavor of the tincture.

Cover the herb with liquid, seal the container, shake up the mixture, and allow the tincture to stand in a warm place (70°–80°F) for two weeks, shaking the container daily. After two weeks, strain out the herbs and filter out any residue. Use under the tongue in drops, take with water or hot tea, or further dilute the tincture in more alcohol.

Penne con Tre Formaggi e Canapa
(Penne with three cheeses and cannabis)

A variation on the classic Italian dish. Cook 1 lb. dried penne or other short pasta in boiling water until *al dente*. While the pasta is cooking, heat 4 tbs. olive oil in a skillet. Add $1/2$ c. chopped cannabis. Cover and saute for 10 minutes. Add 2 tbs. butter and melt. Stir in 3 tbs. flour until smooth. Gradually add 2 c. milk, stirring constantly. When the sauce has reached a velvety texture, stir in 2 c. of mixed grated cheese (parmesan, fontina, and bel paesa is the classic mix, but you can also use cheddar, monterey jack, gruyere, or any other good melting cheese). Drain pasta, pour sauce over pasta, and serve. Serves 4–6.

Root Decoction *(For topical use only)*

Boil the root of a cannabis plant in water, stirring occassionally and crushing up the root as you go. Cook down into a paste. Smear onto wounds, burned or damaged skin, inflamed or aching joints, etc., for analgesic and antibiotic effects.

Cannabis Helper

Select $1/2$ c. of cured bud or shake, and remove as much stem and seed as possible. Chop up and run through a sifter, if desired. In a skillet, melt three tablespoons of butter. Stir in the cannabis powder bit by bit, and sauté at a medium temperature (not too hot), stirring constantly with a spatula to avoid burning. When it takes on a smooth, creamy consistency, fold into any standard recipe. Remember to reduce the amount of flour and oil used in the recipe to compensate for the cannabis helper.

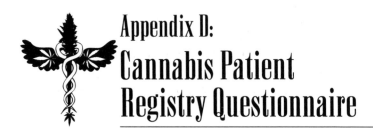

Appendix D:
Cannabis Patient
Registry Questionnaire

Cannabis Patient Registry/CPR
2121 Commonwealth Avenue
Suite 200-G
Charlotte, NC 28205
(704) 334-1798
FAX (704) 334-1799
cpr@maps.org
http://www.maps.org
contact: Sylvia Thyssen

Dear Cannabis Patient Registry Participant,

Welcome to the Cannabis Patient Registry (CPR). Healing Arts Press has included the CPR in *Hemp for Health* so that it can reach the broadest possible audience. The goal of the CPR is to help protect the rights of seriously ill Americans who use cannabis medicinally by creating a network of as many patients as possible. The CPR has been made possible by a grant from the Drug Policy Foundation.

The Cannabis Patient Registry exists to benefit the community of cannabis patients and compassionate caregivers by documenting the widespread medicinal use of cannabis. It will hopefully play a positive role in the effort to influence the scientific and political forces which currently obstruct legal access to medical cannabis.

This questionnaire will take about fifteen minutes for you to complete. Please photocopy it from the back of the book, fill it out, and mail it to us at the above address. Response to it will be kept confidential and the CPR will not give out your name or number to other organizations or to individuals unless you specifically authorize otherwise. The questionnaire is structured around the elements of a medical necessity defense. In the future, the CPR might expand to include additional documentation about your medical history in the form of more detailed questionnaires that track your symptoms and use of cannabis over time.

We urge you to obtain a written note from your physician, on letterhead. It should at least indicate your diagnosis, but may also include whether Marinol or other drugs have been tried, that cannabis provides the best relief, and that the doctor would prescribe it to you if it were legally available. If you have a note from your doctor, please attach a copy of it to this survey once you complete it and return it to the CPR. If you do not yet have a note, we can send you a packet of information that you could give to your physician to inform him or her about aspects of the medical cannabis issue.

If you would be interested in writing a personal account describing your experience with medical cannabis, we are posting such accounts on the Internet (World Wide Web) so as to put a human face on this issue to people all over the world. Such accounts can be anonymous.

Thank you for taking the time to fill out this questionnaire. Please feel free to call if you have questions, suggestions, or comments.

Sincerely,

Sylvia Thyssen

CPR Project Director

CANNABIS PATIENT
REGISTRY PATIENT QUESTIONNAIRE

Personal Use & Medical History

(Your response to this questionnaire will be kept confidential)

Today's date: _____

1. Have you ever or do you currently use cannabis to treat yourself for any of the following medical conditions or symptoms that you have?

	EVER USED	CURRENTLY USE
		(Please circle the main one!)
allergies	____	____
anxiety	____	____
asthma	____	____
cancer (what kind?)	____	____
depression	____	____
diarrhea	____	____
dystonia	____	____
epilepsy	____	____
glaucoma	____	____
HIV/AIDS	____	____
Huntington's chorea	____	____
insomnia	____	____
labor pains	____	____
mania	____	____
manic-depressive disorder	____	____
menstrual cramps	____	____
migraine	____	____
multiple sclerosis	____	____
nausea	____	____
Parkinson's disease	____	____
schizophrenia	____	____
spasticity	____	____
spinal cord injury	____	____
substance abuse	____	____

Tourette's syndrome   ____   ____

tremor   ____   ____

weight loss   ____   ____

vomiting   ____   ____

to reduce use of another medication(s) ____   ____

other condition(s) or symptom(s)   ____   ____

In your words, what medical condition, disease, or symptom do you use cannabis for? Please use extra pages if you need to.

_____

_____

2. Do you also use cannabis for nonmedical purposes?

     _____ yes _____ no _____ I don't differentiate

for what reason(s) do you use it nonmedically?

_____

_____

If you are currently using cannabis medicinally, please skip to question #5. If you used cannabis medicinally in the past, but not currently, please answer questions #3 and #4 first.

3. How long did you use cannabis medicinally in the past?

     _____ (years and/or months)

4. Please check below why you discontinued use and fill in blank where applicable:

_____ I no longer experience the symptoms for which I sought relief because: _____

_____ I found a more effective method of alleviating my symptoms and it is: _____

_____ I experienced health complications from my use of cannabis in the form of: _____

_____ I experienced legal problems from my medical use of cannabis

_____ I can't afford it

_____ there is no available supply

_____ my doctor told me to stop smoking any substance

5. When you use cannabis medicinally, how much do you use?

_____ 6 or more grams per day
_____ 5–6 grams per day
_____ 4–5 grams per day
_____ 3–4 grams per day
_____ 2–3 grams per day
_____ 1–2 grams per day
_____ $^1/_2$–1 gram per day
_____ less than $^1/_2$–1 gram per day
_____ several grams per week
_____ several grams per month
_____ only when I have symptoms, which occurs_____ times per month
_____ OTHER / please list here: _____

_____

_____

6. How do you use cannabis medicinally? Please put a #1 in front of the method you use the most, #2 in front of the method you use the second most frequently, etc. Put a 0 if you have never tried that method.

_____ joint
_____ pipe or bat
_____ water pipe / bong
_____ vaporizer
_____ brownies, cookies, or other foods
_____ tinctures, teas, or other drinks
_____ OTHER / please list here:

7. How did you decide to try cannabis for your condition or symptoms? (check all that apply)

_____ book or article about cannabis
_____ suggestion from a family friend or acquaintance

_____ suggestion from personal physician

_____ I had been a recreational user and I found out by "accident"

_____ other reason / please list here:_____

_____

_____

8. How much money per month do you spend on cannabis?

_____

9. Do you smoke tobacco? _____ yes
(if so, how much _____) _____ no

The following questions ask about other medications you may use or may have tried:

10. What has been your experience with Marinol, the oral THC capsule?

_____ never used

_____ tried it and didn't like it / please list why here:

_____ tried it and thought it worked but stopped using it because: _____

_____ current user with partial relief

_____ current user with complete relief

_____ other:

11. If you have never tried Marinol, would you be willing to try it in comparison to cannabis? _____ yes _____ no

12. If you have tried Marinol or currently use it, which provides better relief? _____ cannabis _____ Marinol

13. Are you currently using any prescription drugs for your condition or symptoms in addition to using cannabis for your condition or symptoms? _____ yes _____ no

If yes, please list the drugs, dose (if you know it), frequency of use (once daily, etc.), and how it works for you (does it work well, or do you like cannabis better, does cannabis help it work better, etc.)

Drug	Dose	Frequency of use	How does it work for you?
_____	_____	_____	_____
_____	_____	_____	_____
_____	_____	_____	_____
_____	_____	_____	_____

These are some of the comments that other patients have given when describing their medications:

"a combination of cannabis and another drug is most effective"

"cannabis helps me to cut down on drugs that give me unpleasant side effects"

"cannabis blocks the side effects of one or more of the drugs I use"

"cannabis helps with some of my symptoms and I use another medicine for other symptoms"

"other drugs do not provide the relief that I get from cannabis"

"cannabis works but I hate to smoke"

Please use this space if you would like to make additional comments on how your use of cannabis compares to or works with your other medicine(s): _____

_____

_____

_____

14. Are there other prescription drugs that you have tried **in the past** for your condition in addition to using cannabis for your condition? ____ yes ____ no

Drug	Dose	Frequency of use	How does it work for you?
_____	_____	_____	_____
_____	_____	_____	_____
_____	_____	_____	_____
_____	_____	_____	_____

15. How much money per month do you spend on other medications? Please estimate your costs plus costs to your insurance company, Medicare, or Medicaid: _____

_____

_____

_____

_____

The following questions ask about your doctor:

16. Does your doctor know that you use cannabis medicinally?
_____ yes _____ no _____ I don't see a doctor

If **yes,** please check all that apply:

My doctor is . . .

_____ strongly discouraging of my use

_____ mildly discouraging of my use

_____ mildly supportive of my use

_____ strongly supportive of my use

_____ the person who recommended that I try cannabis

17. If your doctor does not know you use medicinal cannabis, would you be able to speak with him at some later date?
_____ yes _____ no _____ maybe

18. If your doctor knows you use medicinal cannabis, do you have a letter of support or prescription from him indicating he would prescribe cannabis to you if it were a legally available medicine? _____ yes _____ no
(If so, please include and return a copy of your letter of recommendation or a prescription)

The following questions ask about your involvement with the medical cannabis movement:

18. Are you involved with a grassroots medical cannabis advocacy effort such as a Buyers Club, Green Cross, Cannabis Action Network, etc.? _____ yes _____ no

(If you are working with the medical cannabis movement, we would love to hear about what you're doing. Maybe we could share your good ideas with other activists.)

19. The CPR will not give your name or number to other organizations or to individuals. Would you be interested in receiving information from the CPR about other efforts in the medical cannabis movement? _____ yes _____ no

20. If a patient calls us and would like to be in contact with another patient with your condition or in your geographic area, would you like us to call you to see if you're interested in talking to them? _____ yes _____ no

21. If a reporter calls us and would like to interview a patient with your condition or in your geographic area, would you like us to call you to see if you're interested in talking to them? _____ yes _____ no

22. If we call you and you're not there, is it o.k. to leave a message about why we're calling? _____ yes _____ no

23. May we send mailings to you with the return address: "MAPS/CPR, 2121 Commonwealth Avenue, Suite 200-G, Charlotte NC 28205?" _____ yes _____ no

24. Would you be interested in participating in a more extensive data-gathering project designed to track your symptoms and use of cannabis over time? _____ yes _____ no _____ don't know

Your name: _____

Address: _____

_____

Phone: daytime / _____ evening / _____
    (Feel free to call collect and we can return your call)

(if applicable) Email / _____ Fax / _____

What is your gender: _____ Female _____ Male

What is your age: _____

I am currently _____ working _____ on disability _____ retired
    _____ unemployed _____ a student _____ OTHER:

Feel free to add comments about any of the items on this
    questionnaire or anything else about the CPR. You are
    encouraged to give details about your medical history in
    your own words, particularly if you feel this survey does
    not adequately address your situation.

Thank you for participating in this survey. If you have addi-
    tional questions, please contact Sylvia at: CPR, 2121 Com-
    monwealth Avenue, Suite 200-G, Charlotte NC 28205,
    (704) 334-1798, FAX (704) 334-1799, email:
    cpr@maps.org. I'll be happy to call you right back.

There are issues about your use of cannabis which you might not want to share, but which can help in getting a clearer picture of what the range of experience of medical cannabis users is. Please answer the following questions only if you are comfortable in doing so.

How do you supply yourself with cannabis? Please check all that are applicable.

_____ grow my own

_____ donations from friends or acquaintances

_____ Cannabis Buyers Club

_____ I buy from someone I know

_____ I buy from someone I don't know

_____ other / please explain _____

Have you ever faced legal problems as a result of your medical use of cannabis? _____ yes _____ no

If yes, please check which situation applies to you:
_____ I was arrested, the charges were dropped.
_____ I'm facing trial. Comments: _____

_____
_____ I was convicted and sentenced to: _____

_____
_____ I went to jail.

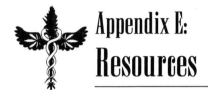

Appendix E:
Resources

RESINOUS CANNABIS:

American Civil
Liberties Union
132 W. 43rd St.
New York, NY 10036
212-944-9800
Legal support for civil liberties violations.

Alliance for Cannabis
Therapeutics
PO Box 21210 Dept. E
Washington, DC 20009
202-483-8595
Fax: 703-354-9695
Medical marijuana information.

Americans for Medical Rights
1250 Sixth St. # 202
Santa Monica, CA 90401
310-394-2952
Fax: 310-451-7494
Coordinating state initiatives for medical rights.

American Public Health
Association
1015 Fifteenth St. NW # 300
Washington, DC 20005
202-789-5600
Fax: 202-789-5661
Adopted a policy in support of medical marijuana.

Business Alliance for
Commerce in Hemp
PO Box 71093
Los Angeles, CA 90071-0093
310-288-4152
Fax: 510-215-8326
ConradBACH@aol.com
*Comprehensive cannabis reform
organization.*

Criminal Justice Policy
 Foundation
1899 L St. NW # 500
Washington, DC 20036
202-835-9075
Fax: 202-833-8561
esterling@igc.apc.org
Drug policy research and support.

Common Sense for
 Drug Policy
3619 Tallwood Terrace
Falls Church, Virginia 22041
703-354-5694
Fax: 703-354-5695
kevzeese@laser.net
*Supports human rights in the
Drug War.*

Drug Policy Foundation
4455 Connecticut Ave. NW
B-500
Washington, DC 20008-2302
202-537-5005
Fax: 202-537-3007
dpf@dpf.org
Drug policy research and support.

Human Rights '95
PO Box 1716
El Cerrito, CA 94530
510-215-8326
Fax: 510-215-8326
MikkiBACH@aol.com
*Prisoner case histories, analysis,
photo exhibit.*

Multidisciplinary Association
for Psychedelic Studies
2121 Commonwealth Avenue
Charlotte, NC 28205-3048
704-334-1798
Fax: 704-334-1799
sylvia@maps.org
http://www.maps.org
*Supports FDA-approved research
on cannabis and psychedelics.*

Marijuana Policy Project
PO Box 77492
Washington, DC 20013
202-462-5747
Fax: 202-232-0442
mpp@mpp.org
http://www.mpp.org
Cannabis reform lobbyists.

National Organization to
Reform Marijuana Laws
1001 Connecticut Ave NW
1010
Washington, DC 20036
202-483-5500
NatlNORML@aol.com
http://www.norml.org
Cannabis reform education &
organization.

INDUSTRIAL HEMP
PRODUCTS, HEMPSEED:

Agricultural Hemp
Association
PO Box 8534
Denver, CO 80201
303-298-7377
Fax: 303-298-7385
ahavoter@aol.com
Spearheading industrial hemp
legislation.

Hemp Industries Association
PO Box 1080
Occidental, CA 95465
707-874-3648
info@thehia.org
http://www.thehia.org
Trade association of hemp
businesses. Call for a listing of
hempseed sources.

International Hemp
Association
Postbus 7500
1070AA Amsterdam, The
Netherlands
Scientific research foundation.

Industrial Hemp Council
PO Box 259329
Madison, WI 53725-9329
608-224-5135
Fax 608-224-5110
sholtea@wheel.datcp.state.wi.us
Industrial hemp advocates.

Notes

Introduction

1. "Deglamorising cannabis," *Lancet* 346 (1995): 1241.
2. *Merck Manual of Diagnosis and Therapy* (Rahway, N.J.: Merck Pharmaceuticals, 1992).
3. L. Grinspoon, "Marihuana as Medicine: A Plea for Reconsideration," *Journal of the American Medical Association* 273 (1995): 1875–76.

Hemp: A Plant for All Seasons

1. Coincidentally, hemp and mulberry were used in China to produce the first paper, circa A.D. 100.
2. J. Lamarck, *Encyclopedia*, vol. 1 (1788), 695.
3. Ruderalis may eventually prove to be a useful source of CBD or other compounds.
4. In tropical zones or in greenhouses, this cycle can be extended for several years. I have seen indoor-grown "mother plants" used for making clones that have been in production for six years or more.
5. Indoor growing techniques using clones can now reduce this length to 1–2 cm.
6. L. Dewey, "Hemp," *Yearbook of the United States Department of Agriculture, 1913.* (Washington, DC: U. S. Government Printing Office, 1914), 286–87.
7. Seed, herbal, and biofuel uses remove more soil nutrients and require more nutrient replacement.
8. 2.5–4 mm (1/10–3/16 in.) thick. 3–6 mm (1/8–1/4 in.) long. Weight: 0.008–0.027 g. Dewey, "Hemp."
9. *Ibid.*
10. This includes balancing the pH level of acidity, and eliminating certain soil pathogens.
11. Based on analysis of government-seized marijuana by the federal Mississippi Potency Monitoring Project, University of Mississippi, marijuana potency is fairly stable. Figures are: 1982, 3.5; 1983, 3.23; 1984, 2.39; 1985, 2.82; 1986, 2.3; 1987, 2.93; 1988, 3.29; 1989, 3.06; 1990, 3.36; 1991, 3.36; 1992, 3.0; 1993, 3.32. The study is sometimes criticized for

focusing on relatively low-grade Mexican cannabis.

12. The ratio of several compounds affects its efficacy, including THC and CBD.

13. E. P. M. de Meijer, "Hemp Variations As Pulp Source Researched in The Netherlands," *Pulp and Paper* (July 1993): 41–43.

14. C. Waller, "Chemistry of Marijuana," *Pharmacological Reviews* 23 (1971): 4.

15. G. Fournier and M.R. Paris, "Le Chanvre Papetier (*Cannabis sativa* L.) Cultive en France: Le Point sur ses Constituants," *Plantes Medicinales et Phytotherapie* 13 (1979): 116–21.

16. J. Beutler and A. Der Marderosian, "Chemotaxonomy of Cannabis I. Cross-breeding Between Cannabis Sativa and C. Ruderalis, with Analysis of Cannabinoid Content," *Economic Botany* 32 (1978): 387–394.

17. W. Booth, "Marijuana Receptor Exists In Brain, Study Confirms," *Washington Post* (August 9, 1990).

18. H. van der Werf, *Crop Physiology of Fibre Hemp* (Wageningen, The Netherlands: Proefschrift Wageningen, 1994).

Cannabis Through the Millennia

1. T. Mikuriya, *Marijuana: Medical Papers, 1839–1972* (Oakland, CA: MediComp Press, 1973).

2. R. Mechoulam, *Cannabinoids as Therapeutic Agents* (Boca Raton, FL: CRC Press, 1986).

3. N. Patnaik, *The Garden of Life: An Introduction to the Healing Plants of India* (New York, NY: Doubleday Books, 1993), 8.

4. Dioscorides, *Materia Medica*, 3.165.

5. *Anicia Juliana*, 512.

6. Caius Plinius Secundus, *De Historia Natura*, 20.97.

7. C. Galen, *De Facultatibus Alimentorum*, 100.49.

8. K. Jones, *Nutritional and Medicinal Guide to Hemp Seed* (Gib-sons, BC: Rainforest Botanical Laboratory, 1995), 15–19.

9. E. Abel, *Marihuana: The first 12,000 years* (New York: Plenum Press, 1980), 139–40.

10. G. Da Orta, *Colloquies on the Simples and Drugs of India, 1563*, Henry Southern, trans. (London, 1913).

11. Abel, *Marihuana*, 119.

12. N. Culpeper, *Complete Herbal* (London: Richard Evans Co., 1814), 91.

13. J. J. Moreau, "Lypemanie avec Stupeur: Tendence á la demence, Traitement par l'extrait Guerison, Resineux de Cannabis indica," *Gazette des Hopitaux Civils et Militaires* 30 (1857): 391.

14. W. B. O'Shaughnessy, "On the Preparation of Indian Hemp, or Gunjah," *Translations of the Medical and Physical Society of Calcutta* (1842): 421–461.

15. He gave some cannabis to Peter Squire, whose pharmacy began to prepare Squires Extract.
16. G. B. Wood and F. Bache, *Dispensatory of the United States* (Philadelphia, PA: Lippincott, Brambo and Co., 1854), 339.
17. J. R. Reynolds, "On the Therapeutical Uses and Toxic Effects of Cannabis Indica," *Lancet* 1 (1890): 637–38.
18. M. Sassman, "Cannabis Indica in Pharmaceuticals," *Journal of the Medical Society of New Jersey* 35 (1938): 51–52.
19. Cases of multiple drug users intravenously injecting boiled suspensions of cannabis were followed by severe problems. Chills, muscle aches, weakness, abdominal cramps, slowed respiratory rate, and low blood pressure were uniformly observed. Other patients experienced diarrhea, vomiting, very rapid pulse, elevated body temperature, enlarged spleen and liver, pulmonary congestion, and abnormal kidney function in reaction to the intravenous injection of plant material. Don't do it! See N. E. Gary and V. Keylon, "Intravenous administration of marihuana," *Journal of the American Medical Association* 11 (1970): 501.
20. Du Pont, *Annual Report*, 1937.
21. L. Du Pont, "From Test Tube to You," *Popular Mechanics* (June 1939): 805.
22. Senate Committee on Finance, *Hearing on HR 6906* (July 12, 1937).
23. Department of Health, Education and Welfare, *Marihuana and Health, A Report to Congress from the Secretary* (March, 1971), 54.
24. R. S. El-Mallakh, "Marijuana and Migraine," (Farmington, CT: University of Connecticut Health Center, Dept. of Neurology, 1987).
25. A. T. Weil, N. E. Zinberg, and J. M. Nelsen, "Clinical and Psychological Effects of Marihuana in Man," *Science* 162 (1968): 1234–42; L. D. Chait, "Delta-9 THC Content and Human Marijuana Self-administration," (Chicago, IL: Pritzker School of Medicine, University of Chicago, 1989).
26. K. Green and T. F. McDonald, "Ocular Toxicology of Marijuana: Update," *Journal of Toxicology* 6 (1987): 239–382; R. Hepler and R. Petrus, "Experiences with Administration of Marijuana to Glaucoma Patients," *The Pharmacology of Marijuana*, Braude and Szara, eds. (New York: Raven Press), 63–94.
27. L. E. Hollister, "Hunger and Appetite after Single Doses of Marihuana, Ethanol and Dextroamphetamine," *Clinical Pharmacology and Therapeutics* (1971); R. C. Randall, *Cancer Treatment and Marijuana Therapy* (Washington, DC: Galen Press, 1990).
28. Sallan, et al., "Antiemetics in Patients Receiving Chemotherapy for Cancer," *New England Journal of Medicine* 302 (1980): 135.
29. V. Vinciguerra, T. Moore, and E. Brennan, "Inhalation Marijuana as an Antiemetic for Cancer Chemotherapy," *NY State Journal of Medicine* 88 (1988): 525–27.

30. R. Doblin and M. Kleiman, "Marihuana as Anti-emetic Medicine: A Survey of Oncologists' Attitudes and Experiences," *Journal of Clinical Oncology* (1991): 1275–80.

31. G. Fournier, et al., "Identification of a New Chemotype in Cannabis sativa: Cannabigerol Dominant Plants, Biogenetic and Agronomic Prospects," *Planta Medica* 53 (1987): 277–80; S. Cohen, *Therapeutic Potential of Marijuana's Components*, American Council on Marijuana and Other Psychoactive Drugs (1982); E. A. Formukong, A. T. Evans, and F. J. Evans, "Analgesic and Anti-inflammatory Activity of Constituents of *Cannabis sativa* L.," *Inflammation* 12 (1988): 361–71; Consroe, et al., "Open Label Evaluation of Cannabidiol in Dystonic Movement Disorders," *International Journal of Neuroscience* 30 (1986): 277–82; J. M. Cunha, et al., "Chronic Administration of Cannabidiol to Healthy Volunteers and Epileptic Patients," *Pharmacology* 21 (1980): 175–85; Meinck, Schonle, and Conrad, "Effect of Cannabinoids on Spasticity and Ataxia in MS," *Journal of Neurology* 236 (1989): 120–22; Sandyk, et al., "Effects of Cannabidiol in Huntington's Disease," *Neurology* 36 (1986): 342.

32. I. G. Karniol and E. A. Carlini, "Pharmacological Interaction between Cannabidiol and Δ 9-THC," *Psycho-pharmacologia* 33 (1973): 53–70; I. G. Karniol, et al., "Cannabidiol Interferes with the Effects of delta 9-THC in Man," *European Journal of Pharmacy* 28 (1974): 172–77.

33. A.W. Zuardi, et al., "Effects of Cannabidiol in Animal Models Predictive of Anti-psychotic Activity," *Psychopharmacology* 104 (1991): 260–64.

34. Mechoulam and Feigenbaum, "Progress towards Cannabinoid Drugs," *Medicinal Chemistry* 2 (1987): 159–207.

Sympathetic Health-Care Systems

1. M. A. Weiner and J. Weiner, *Herbs That Heal* (Mill Valley, CA: Quantum Books, 1994), 225–26.

2. C. Bennet, L. Osburn, and J. Osburn, *Green Gold and the Tree of Life: Marijuana in Magic and Religion* (Frazier Park, CA: Access Unlimited, 1995), 102, 104, 105, 108, 144.

3. E. M. Brecher and the editors of Consumer Reports, *Licit and Illicit Drugs: The Consumers Union Report* (New York: Little, Brown and Co., 1972), 397–98.

4. J. Zand, R. Walton, and B. Roundtree, *Smart Medicine for a Healthier Child* (Garden City Park, NY: Avery, 1994), 73–75, 432–34.

5. One possible problem and a common criticism of homeopathy is that, rather than treating the underlying condition, it might serve to mask certain symptoms, thus making accurate diagnosis more difficult.

6. J. Kleijnen, P. Knipschild, and G. ter Riet, "Clinical trials of homeopathy," *British Medical Journal* 302 (1991): 316.

7. G. H. G. Jahr, *New Homeopathic Pharmacopoeia and Posology of the Preparation*

of Homeopathic Medicines (Philadelphia, PA: J. Dobson, 1842), 137.

8. W. Boericke, *Homeopathic Materia Medica: Comprising the Characteristic and Guiding Symptoms of the Remedies* (Irthlingborough, England: Woolnough Bookbinding Ltd., 1987), 160–62.

9. B. Dash, *Fundamentals of Ayurvedic Medicine*, 4th ed. (New Delhi, India: Bansal and Co., 1984), ix–xvi, 141–57. Chapters 7 and 8 deal with three popular ayurvedic drugs: cannabis, garlic, and haritaki (*Terminalia chebula* Retz). Ayurvedic texts describe them as products of *amrita* (ambrosia). Cannabis is also used as a psychotropic agent.

10. *Atharva Veda*, xi, 8(6) 15.

11. In Satya yuga, it was white; in Treta yuga, red; in Dvapara yuga, yellow; and in Kali yuga, green.

12. Brahamana type plant is white; Ksatriya, red; Vaisya, green; and Sudra, black.

13. Four different types of mantras have been prescribed in *Sri Kali Nityarcana* for purification of different types of cannabis.

14. Janmausadhi-mantra-tapah-samadhijah siddhayah, *Yoga Sutra* IV: I.

15. *Susruta samhita,* sutra 15:41.

16. *Srikali Nityarcana* (1955).

17. *Panini,* v, 2.29.

18. *Anandakanda* (1952), 236.

19. Designated at one, three, five, six, nine, ten, eleven, or thirteen leaflets in a set, *Anandakanda*, 236.

20. Cannabis obtained from the male plant and the pollinated female plant is commonly known as *bhang.* That obtained from the virgin female plant is called *ganja,* and is stronger than bhang. Charas is the resin collected from living plants.

21. One recipe mentions that the medicine should first be offered to Lords Shiva, Indra, Kamadeva, and Gananatha, and thereafter it should be offered to Fire, while reciting a mantra. Dash, *Fundamentals of Ayurvedic Medicine.*

22. A tropical disease characterized by anemia, gastrointestinal disorders, sore throat, etc.; psilosis.

23. Dash, *Fundamentals of Ayurvedic Medicine.*

24. *Susruta samhita,* Kalpa 15:5.

25. In *Anandakanda* a complete chapter is devoted to the description of cannabis and how to process it for therapeutic rejuvenation. Also see Dash, *Fundamentals of Ayurvedic Medicine,* 147–48.

26. *Mahabharata,* I 76, 43–68.

The Cannabinoids

1. M. A. ElSohly, et al., "Constituents of *Cannabis saiva* L. XXIV: The potency of confiscated marijuana, hashish and hash oil over a 10-year

period," *Journal of Forensic Sciences* 29 (1984).

2. R. C. Clarke and D. W. Pate, "Medical Marijuana," *Journal of the International Hemp Association* 1 (1994): 9–12.

3. Christensen, et al., *Science* 172 (1971): 165.

4. E. P. M. de Meijer, "Characterization of Cannabis Accessions with Regard to Cannabinoid Content in Relation to Other Plant Characters," *Euphytica* 62 (1992): 187–200.

5. G. Fournier, et al., "Identification of a New Chemotype in Cannabis sativa: Cannabigerol Dominant Plants, Biogenetic and Agronomic Prospects," 277–80.

6. R. P. Latta and B. J. Eaton, "Seasonal Fluctuations in Cannabinoid Content of Kansas Marijuana," *Economic Botany* 29 (1975): 153–63.

7. Mechoulam and Feigenbaum, "Progress Towards Cannabinoid Drugs," 159–207.

8. Thanks to Eric Skidmore for helping research this information.

9. Formukong, Evans, and Evans, "Analgesic and Anti-Inflammatory Activity of Constituents of Cannabis sativa L."

10. I. G. Karniol and E. A. Carlini, "Pharmacological Interaction between CBD and Δ-9-THC," *Psychopharmacologia* 33 (1973): 53–70.

11. Karniol, et al., "Cannabidiol Interferes with the Effects of THC in Man," *European Journal of Pharmacology* 28 (1974): 172–77.

12. A. W. Zuardi, et al., "Action of Cannabidiol on the Anxiety and Other Effects Produced by Δ9–THC in Normal Subjects," *Psychopharacology* 76 (1982): 245–50.

13. J. M. Cunha, et al., "Chronic Administration of Cannabidiol to Healthy Volunteers and Epileptic Patients," *Pharmacology* 21 (1980): 175–85; Consroe, et al., "Open Label Evaluation," 277–82; Sandyk, et al., "Effects of CBD in Huntington's Disease," 342; Formukong, Evans, and Evans, "Analgesic and Anti-inflammatory Activity of Constituents of *Cannabis sativa* L.," 361–71; M. Carlini, et al., "Possivel Efeito Hipnotico do Cannabidiol no ser Humano," *Ciencia e Cultura* 31 (1979): 315–22; Zuardi, Rodrigues, and Cunha, "Effects of CBD in Animal Models Predictive of Anti-psychotic Activity," 260–64.

14. Formukong, Evans, and Evans, "Analgesic and Anti-inflammatory Activity of Constituents of *Cannabis sativa* L.," 361–71.

15. Consroe, et al., "Open Label Evaluation" 277–82.

16. Sandyk, et al., "Effects of CBD in Huntington's Disease," 342.

17. Cunha, et al., "Chronic Administration of CBD to Healthy Volunteers and Epileptic Patients," 175–85.

18. E. A. Carlini and J. A. Cunha, "Hypnotic and Anti-epileptic Effects of CBD," *Journal of Clinical Pharmacology* 21 (1981): 417S–427S.

19. Zuardi, Rodrigues, and Cunha, "Effects of CBD in Animal Models Predictive of Anti-psychotic Activity," 260–64.

20. Sandyk and Awerbuch, "Marijuana and Tourette's Syndrome," *Journal of Clinical Psycho Pharmacology* 8 (1988): 444–45; Conti, et al., "Antidyskinetic Effects of Cannabidiol," *Proceedings of the International Congress on Marijuana* (Melbourne, Australia, 1987).

Marijuana Classification

1. The 1969 ruling by the Supreme Court in Timothy Leary's case that applying for a tax stamp to handle an illegal substance was unconstitutional self-incrimination forced some revisions to the law at the time that early proselytizers for LSD were active. When hallucinogens were added to the index, marijuana was transferred to that category.
2. H. Isbell and D. R. Jasinski, "A Comparison of LSD-25 with Δ-9-THC and Attempted Cross Tolerance between LSD and THC," *Psychopharmacologia* 14 (1969): 115–23; Isbell, et al., "Effects of Δ-9-THC in Man," *Psychopharmacologia* 11 (1967): 184–88; L. D. Clark, R. Hughes, and E. N. Nakashima, "Behavioral Effects of Marihuana: Experimental Studies," *Archives of General Psychiatry* 23 (1970): 193–98; Melges, et al., "Marihuana and temporal disintegration," *Science* 168 (1970): 1118–20.
3. L. E. Hollister and F. Moore, "Urinary Catecholamine Excretion Following LSD in Man," *Psychopharmacologia* 11 (1967): 270; Melges, et al., "Marihuana and Temporal Disintegration," 1118–20.
4. L. E. Hollister, "Steroids and Moods: Correlations in Schizophrenics and Subjects Treated with LSD, Mescaline, THC, and Synhexyl," *Journal of Clinical Pharmacology* 9 (1969): 24–29; L. E. Hollister, R. K. Richards, and H. K. Gillespie, "Comparison of THC and Synhexyl in Man," *Clinical Pharmacology and Therapeutics* 9 (1968): 783–91; L. E. Hollister and F. Moore, "Urinary Catecholamine Excretion Following Mescaline in Man," 2015.
5. Isbell and Jasinski, "A Comparison of LSD-25 with Δ-9-THC and Attempted Cross Tolerance between LSD and THC," 115–23.
6. L. E. Hollister, S. L. Sherwood, and A. Cavasino, "Marihuana and the Human Electroencephalogram," *Pharmacological Research Communications* 1971; R. Jones and G. Stone, "Psychological Studies of Marijuana and Alcohol in Man," *Psychopharmacologia* 18 (1970): 108–17; E. Rodin, E. F. Domino, and J. P. Porzak, "The Marihuana-induced 'Social High'— Neurological and Electroencephalographic Concomitants," *JAMA* 213 (1970): 1300–1302.
7. Brill, et al., "The Marijuana Problems. UCLA Interdepartmental Conference," *Annals of Internal Medicine* 73 (1970): 449–65.
8. L. E. Hollister, "Hunger and Appetite after Single Doses of Marihuana, Ethanol and Dextroamphetamine," *Clinical Pharmacology and Therapeutics* (1972); L. E. Hollister and H. K. Gillespie, "Marihuana, Ethanol

and Dextroamphetamine: Mood and Mental Function Alterations," *Archives of General Psychiatry* 23 (1970): 199-203; R. Jones and G. Stone, "Psychological Studies of Marijuana and Alcohol in Man," 108–117; J. E. Manno, "Clinical Investigations with Marihuana and Alcohol" (unpublished paper, Indiana University, 1970).

9. J. M. Ritchie, *The Pharmacological Basis of Therapeutics,* Goodman and Gilman, eds., 3rd ed. (New York: Macmillan Company, 1965), 143–53.

10. Hollister and Gillespie, "Marihuana, Ethanol and Dextroamphetamine; Mood and Mental Function Alterations," 199–203; Hollister, "Hunger and Appetite after Single Doses of Marihuana, Ethanol and Dextroamphetamine."

11. Jones and Stone, "Psychological Studies of Marijuana and Alcohol in Man," 108–17.

12. Ohlsson, et al., "Plasma Δ-9-THC Concentrations and Clinical Effects after Oral and Intravenous Administration and Smoking," *Clinical Pharmacology Therapeutics* 28 (1980): 409.

13. Peat, Jones, et al., "The Disposition of Δ-9-THC . . . In frequent and Infrequent Marijuana Users," *Journal of Pharmacol. Exp. Therap.* (1987).

The Resinant Brain

1. M. Leveritt, "Reefer Madness; While Courts Send Users to Prison, Scientists . . . Find Little to Support Dangers of Pot," *Arkansas Times* (Sept. 16, 1993): 11.

2. R. Mestel, "Cannabis: The Brain's Other Supplier," *New Scientist* (July 31, 1993).

3. L. Wallach, "The Chemistry of Reefer Madness," *Omni* (August, 1989): 18.

4. R. Mechoulam, Interview by David Pate. *Journal of the International Hemp Association* 1 (1994): 21–23.

5. Johnson, et al., "Selective and Potent Analgesics Derived from Cannabinoids," *Journal of Clinical Pharmacology* 21 (1981): 271S–282S; D. B. Clifford, "Tetrahydrocannabinol for Tremor in Multiple Sclerosis," *Annals of Neurology* 13 (1983): 669–71.

6. H. Meinck, P. W. Schonle, and B. Conrad, "Effect of Cannabinoids on Spasticity and Ataxia in Multiple Sclerosis," *Journal of Neurology* 230 (1989): 120–22.

7. D. Petro and C. Ellenberger, "Treatment of Human Spasticity with delta-9-Tetrahydrocannabinol," *Journal of Clinical Pharmacology* 21 (1981): 413S–416S.

8. H. A. Hare, *Practical Therapeutics* (Philadelphia, 1922), 181.

9. Malec, Harvey, and Cayner, "Cannabis' Effect on Spasticity in Spinal Cord Injury," *Archive of Physical and Medical Rehab* 35 (1982): 198.

10. Cunha, et al., "Chronic Administration of CBD to Healthy Volunteers

and Epileptic Patients," 175–85; D. Feeney, "Marijuana Use Among Epileptics," *JAMA* 235 (1976): 1105; R. Karler and S. A. Turkanis, "The Cannabinoids as Potential Antiepileptics," *Journal of Clinical Pharmacology* 21 (1981): 437S–448S.

11. Maurer, et al., "Delta-9-THC Shows Antispastic and Analgesic Effects in a Single Case Double-Blind Trial," *European Archive of Psychiatry and Clinical Neuroscience* 240 (1990): 1–4.

12. H. A. Hare, *Practical Therapeutics,* 181.

13. S. Benet, "Early Diffusion and Folk Uses of Hemp," *Cannabis and Culture,* V. Rubin, ed. (The Hague, Netherlands: Mouton, 1975), 43, 46.

14. "20 drops gelsemium tincture in full dose, followed by 10–20 drops active fluid extract of cannabis. After this, the patient should be watched, lest he suffer from depression." H. A. Hare, *Practical Therapeutics,* 181.

15. W. E. Dixon, The Pharmacology of Cannabis indica," *British Medical Journal* (Nov. 11, 1897): 1354–57.

16. S. Allentuck and K. M. Bowman, "The Psychiatric Aspects of Marihuana Intoxication," *American Journal of Psychiatry* 99 (1942): 248–51.

17. G. T. Stockings, "A New Euphoriant for Depressive Mental States," *British Medical Journal* (1947): 918–22.

18. Kotin, Post, and Goodwin, "Delta-9 THC in Depressed Patients," *Archives of General Psychiatry* 28 (1973): 345–48.

19. L. Grinspoon and J. B. Bakalar, *Marijuana: The Forbidden Medicine* (New Haven, CT: Yale University Press, 1993): 124–26.

20. J. R. Hubbard, *Investigation of marijuana use across psychiatric diagnosis,* U.S. Dept. of Veterans Affairs, Research and development information system. Project data sheet RCS 100159 (March 1, 1995).

21. Zuardi, et al., "Effects of Cannabidiol in Animal Models Predictive of Anti-Psychotic Activity," 260–64.

22. L. Sloman, *The History of Marijuana in America: Reefer Madness* (Indianapolis, IN: Bobbs-Merrill Company, Inc., 1979): 152–58.

23. Grinspoon and Bakalar, *Marijuana,* 124–26.

24. T. H. Mikuriya, "Cannabis Substitution, an Adjunctive Therapeutic Tool in the Treatment of Alcoholism," *Medical Times* 98 (1970): 187–91.

25. C. K. Himmelsbach, "Treatment of the Morphine Abstinence Syndrome with a Synthetic Cannabis-Like Compound," *Southern Medical Journal* 37 (1944): 26–29.

Sight for Sore Eyes

1. M. W. Adler and E. B. Geller, "Ocular Effects of Cannabinoids," R. Mechoulam, ed., *Cannabinoids as Therapeutic Agents* (Boca Raton, FL: CRC Press, 1986): 51–70.

2. S. Cohen, "Therapeutic Aspects," *Marihuana,* NIDA monograph (Washington, DC, 1976), 194–225.

3. K. Green and T. F. McDonald, "Ocular Toxicology of Marijuana: Update," *Journal of Toxicology* 6 (1987): 239–382.
4. Grinspoon and Bakalar, *Marijuana.*
5. F. L. Young, *In the Matter of Marijuana Rescheduling Petition,* Docket no 86–22 (Sept. 6, 1988).
6. J. E. Manno, et al., "Comparative Effects of Smoking Marihuana and Motor and Mental Performance in Humans," *Clinical Pharmacology and Therapeutics* 11 (1970): 808–15.
7. J. E. Manno, "Clinical Investigations with Marihuana and Alcohol."
8. Weil, Zinberg, and Nelsen, "Clinical and Psychological Effects of Marihuana in Man," 1234–42.
9. D. F. Caldwell, S. A. Myers, and E. F. Domino, "Effects of Marihuana Smoking on Sensory Thresholds in Man," *Psychotomimetic Drugs,* D. Efron, ed. (New York: Raven Press, 1970), 299–321; Caldwell, et al., "Auditory and Visual Threshold Effects of Marihuana in Man," 755–59; Addendum, *Perceptual and Motor Skills* 29 (1969): 922.
10. W. Mayer-Gross, et al., *Clinical Psychiatry* (London: Cassell, 1969); Mayor's Committee on Marihuana, *The Marihuana Problem in the City of New York: Sociological, Medical, Psychological and Pharmacological Studies* (Lancaster, PA: Cattell Press, 1944).
11. R. S. Hepler, I. M. Frank, and J. T. Ungerleider, "The Effects of Marijuana Smoking on Pupillary Size," *American Journal of Opthalmology* (1971).
12. Brill, et al., "The Marijuana Problems. UCLA Interdepartmental Conference," 449–65; Frank, et al., "Marihuana, Tobacco and Functions Affecting Driving," Paper presented at American Psychiatric Association Annual Meeting. (Washington, D. C.: May 1971).
13. He joined a night fishing crew and studied how they navigated without lights in treacherous waters. M. E. West, *Nature* (July 1991); "Marijuana may aid night vision," *Los Angeles Times* (July 1, 1991).
14. I. C. Chopra and R. N. Chopra, "The Use of the Cannabis Drugs in India." *UN Bulletin on Narcotics* 9 (1957): 4–29.
15. F. Ames, "A Clinical and Metabolic Study of Acute Intoxication with Cannabis Sativa and its Role in the Model Psychoses," *Journal of Mental Sciences* 104 (1958): 972–99; Isbell, et al., "Studies on THC," *Bulletin: Problems of Drug Dependence* (Washington, D. C.: Committee on Problems of Drug Dependence, National Academy of Sciences, 1967), 4832-46; S. Allentuck and K. M. Bowman, "The Psychiatric Aspects of Marihuana Intoxication," *American Journal of Psychiatry* 99 (1942): 248–51.
16. Rx—Tincture nucis vomicæ, f3ij (8.0); Tincture cannabis, f3ij (8.0). — M. S.—15 drops (1.0), in water, twice or thrice a day. de Schweinitz. In Hare, *Practical Therapeutics,* 181.

Eating and Digestion

1. Benet, "Early Diffusion and Folk Uses of Hemp," 43, 46.
2. S. E. Sallan, et al., "Antiemetics in Patients Receiving Chemotherapy for Cancer," *New England Journal of Medicine* 302 (1980): 135–38; S. E. Sallan, N. E. Zinberg, and E. Frei, "Antiemetic Effect of Δ-9-THC in Patients Receiving Cancer Chemotherapy," *New England Journal of Medicine* 293 (1975): 795–97.
3. Nelson, et al., "A Phase II Study of Δ-9-THC for Appetite Stimulation in Cancer-Associated Anorexia," *Journal of Palliative Care* 10 (1994): 14–18.
4. R. Doblin and M. Kleiman, "Marihuana as Anti-emetic Medicine: A Survey of Oncologists' Attitudes and Experiences." *Journal of Clinical Oncology* (1991): 1275–80; R. Ostrow, "48% of Cancer Specialists in Study Would Prescribe Pot," *Los Angeles Times* (May 1, 1991).
5. V. Vinciguerra, T. Moore, and E. Brennan, "Inhalation Marijuana as an Antiemetic for Cancer Chemotherapy," *NY State Journal of Medicine* (1988): 525–57.
6. Case History, *Human Rights 95: Atrocities of the Drug War.*
7. L. S. Harris, A. E. Munson, and R. A. Carchman, "Antitumor Properties of Cannabinoids," *The Pharmacology of Marihuana,* Braude and Szara, eds. (New York: Raven, 1976), vol. 2, 773–76.
8. S. J. Bell, *Positive Nutrition for HIV Infection and AIDS* (Chronimed Publishing, 1996).
9. F. Ames, "A Clinical and Metabolic Study of Acute Intoxication with Cannabis Sativa and Its Role in the Model Psychoses," *Journal of Mental Sciences* 104 (1958): 972–99.
10. E. Lindemann, "The Neuro-Physiological Effects of Intoxicating Drugs," *American Journal of Psychiatry* 90 (1933–1934): 1007–1037; Mayor's Committee on Marihuana, *The Marihuana Problem in the City of New York*; Hollister, "Hunger and Appetite After Single Doses of Marihuana, Ethanol and Dextroamphetamine"; Weil, Zinberg, and Nelsen, "Clinical and Psychological Effects of Marihuana in Man," 1234–42; C. J. Miras, "Some aspects of cannabis action," *Hashish: Its Chemistry and Pharmacology,* G. E. W. Wolsten-holme and J. Knight, eds., (London: Ciba Foundation, 1965).
11. Hollister, "Hunger and Appetite After Single Doses of Marihuana, Ethanol and Dextroamphetamine."

Cardiovascular and Pulmonary Systems

1. Ohlsson, et al., "Plasma Δ-9-THC concentrations and clinical effects after oral and intravenous administration and smoking," *Clinical Pharmacology and Therapy* 28 (1980): 409.
2. Isbell, et al., "Studies on THC," 4832–46; R. E. Meyer, et al., "Administration of Marihuana to Heavy and Casual Users," Paper presented at American Psychiatric Association Meeting (Washington, D. C.: May 1971).

3. Crancer, et al., "Simulated driving performance," *Science* 164 (1969): 851–54; Domino, E. F. "Human Pharmacology of Marihuana Smoking," *Journal of Clinical Pharmacology Therapeutics* (1971); Hollister, Richards, and Gillespie, "Comparison of THC and Synhexyl in Man," 783–91; Manno, et al., "Comparative Effects of Smoking Marihuana and Motor and Mental Performance in Humans," 808–15; Mayor's Committee on Marihuana, *The Marihuana Problem in the City of New York;* Waskow, et al., "Psychological Effects of THC," *Review of General Psychiatry* 22 (1970): 97–107; Weil, Zinberg, and Nelsen, "Clinical and Psychological Effects of Marihuana in Man," 1234–42. While smoked doses of 4 and 15 mg THC caused pulse rate increases averaging 22 and 34 beats per minute, respectively, oral doses of 8 and 34 mg produced respective increases of 18 and 33 beats per minute. The two studies used doses up to 70 mg Δ9-THC and an extract containing 255 mg.

4. Cone, Welch, and Lange, "Clonidine Partially Blocks the Physiologic Effects but not the Subjective Effects Produced by Smoking Marijuana," *Pharmacology, Biochemistry and Behavior* 29 (1988): 649–652

5. Dixon, "The Pharmacology of Cannibis indica."

6. Hare, *Practical Therapeutics*, 181. Up to 5 drams of 3 fluid extract, equivalent to 10 minims to man, injected into the jugular vein of a small dog did not produce death.

7. Tobacco is a vasoconstrictor.

8. V. Sim, "Proceedings of a Workshop on Psychotomimetic Drugs," *Psychotomimetic Drugs*, D. Efron., ed. (New York: Raven Press, 1970).

9. 15–70 mg THC or 50–150 mg synhexyl. Hollister, "Steroids and Moods: Correlations in Schizophrenics and Subjects Treated with LSD, Mescaline, THC, and Synhexyl," 24–29; Hollister, Richards, and Gillespie, "Comparison of THC and Synhexyl in Man," 783–91.

10. Mayor's Committee on Marihuana, *The Marihuana Problem in the City of New York.*

11. J. D. P. Graham, "The Bronchodilator Action of Cannabinoids," *Cannabinoids as therapeutic agents*, R. Mechoulam, ed. (Boca Raton, FL: CRC Press, 1986), 147–58.

12. D. Cooley, ed., "After-40 Health and Medical Guide," *Better Homes and Gardens* (1980): 24.

13. D. P. Tashkin, B. J. Shapiro, and I. A. Frank, "Acute Pulmonary Physiologic Effects of Smoked Marihuana and Oral Δ-9-THC in Healthy Young Men," *New England Journal of Medicine* 289 (1973): 336–41; Tashkin, et al., "Effects of Smoked Marihuana in Experimentally Induced Asthma," *American Review of Respiratory Disease* 112 (1975): 377–86.

14. Case history, *Human Rights 95: Atrocities of the Drug War.*

15. P. E. G. Mann, T. N. Finley, and A. J. Ladman, "Marihuana Smoking: a Study of Its Effects on Alveolar Lining Material and Pulmonary

Macrophages Recovered by Bronchopulmonary Lavage," *Journal of Clinical Investigations* (1970): 60a–61a.

16. Hare, *Practical Therapeutics*, 181.

Reproduction, Metabolism, and Topical Applications

1. J. P. Purvis, *Through Uganda to Mt. Elgon* (London: Fisher Unwin, 1909), 336–37.

2. C. Leger and G. Nahas, "Kinetics of Cannabinoid Distribution and Storage with Special Reference to Brain and Testes," *Journal of Clinical Pharmacology* (1981).

3. J. Zias, et al., "Early medical use of cannabis," *Nature* 363 (1993): 215.

4. J. M. Watt and M. G. Breyer-Brandwijk, *The Medicinal and Poisonous Plants of Southern Africa* (Edinburgh: E&S Livingstone, 1932).

5. N. Goundry, trans., *Da Ma. Translations from the Ben Cao Gang Mu* (Madeira Park, B.C., 1995).

6. G.B.Wood and F. Bache, *Dispensatory of the United States* (Philadelphia, PA: Lippincott, Brambo and Co., 1854), 339.

7. R. Batho, "Cannabis Indica," *British Medical Journal* (1883): 1002.

8. E. Abel, *Marihuana.*

9. "Women of Atala capture men and induce them to drink an intoxicating beverage made with cannabis indica. This potion endows the men with great sexual prowess, of which the women take advantage for enjoyment. A woman will enchant him with attractive glances, intimate words, smiles of love and then embraces. In this way she induces him to enjoy sex with her to her full satisfaction. Because of his increased sexual power, the man thinks himself stronger than 10,000 elephants and considers himself almost perfect." *Bhagavat-puran*, 5:24:16.

10. A. Gottlieb, *Sex, Drugs and Aphrodisiacs* (Berkeley, CA: 20th Century Alchemy, 1973), 1993.

11. W. E. Dixon, "The Pharmacology of Cannabis indica," 1354–57.

12. G. Biernson, "Data on Storage of Marijuana in the Body," *Drug Awareness Information Newsletter* (March 1988).

13. J. P. Morgan, "Marijuana Metabolism in the Context of Urine Testing," 107–15.

14. Peat, et. al., "The disposition of Δ-9-THC."

15. Lemberger, et al., "Marihuana: Studies on the Disposition and Metabolism of Δ-9-THC in Man," *Science* 170 (1970): 1320–22.

16. J. P. Morgan, Marijuana Metabolism in the Context of Urine Testing," 107–15.

17. J. Navrátil, "Effectiveness of C. indica in Chronic Otitis Media" (in Czech) *Acta. Univ. Palack.* 6 (1955): 8; J. Jubácek, "A Study of the Effect of C. indica in Oto-rhinolaryngology" (in Czech) *Acta. Univ. Palack.* 6 (1955): 83; J. Jubácek, "A Contribution to the Treatment of Sinusitis

Maxillaris" (in Czech) *Acta. Univ. Palack.* (1961): 207; S. Cohen, "Marijuana as Medicine," *Psychology Today* (1978): 60.

18. L. Ferenczy, L. Gracza, and I. Jakobey, "An Antibacterial Preparation from Hemp (*Cannabis sativa* L.)" (in German) *Naturwissenschaften* 45 (1958): 188; J. Kabelik, Z. Krejci, and F. Santavy, "Cannabis as a Medicament," *UN Bulletin on Narcotics* 12 (1960): 5-23; Z. Krejci, "On the Problem of Substances with Antibacterial Action: Cannabis Effect," *Casopis Lekaru Ceskych.* 43 (1961): 1351–54; A. Radosevic, M. Kupinic, and L. Grlic, "Antibiotic Activity of Various Types of Cannabis Resin," *Nature* 195: 1007–1009.

19. P. Lansky, "Marijuana as Medicine?" *Health World* (February 1991): 46–49.

20. Lancz, et al., "Interaction of Δ-9-THC with Herpes Viruses and Cultural Conditions Associated with Drug-Induced Anti-Cellular Effects," *Drugs of Abuse, Immunity and Imunodeficiency*, H. Friedman, et al., eds. (New York: Plenum Press, 1991), 287–304; Lancz, Specter, and Brown, "Suppressive Effect of Δ-9-THC on Herpes Simplex Cirus Infectivity In Vitro, *Proceedings of the Society for Experimental Biology and Medicine* 196 (1991): 401–404.

21. L. S. Harris, A. E. Munson, and R. A. Carchman, "Antitumor Properties of Cannabinoids," *The Pharmacology of Marihuana*, Braude and Szara, eds., (New York: Raven Press), vol. 2, 773–76.

22. Herodotus. *Histories IV.* 450 B.C. (Cambridge, MA: University Press, 1906), 74–76.

23. R. S. Lees and M. Karel, eds., *Omega-6 Essential Fatty Acids in Health and Disease* (New York: Marcel Dekker, 1990).

24. *Encyclopaedia Britannica*, "hemp."

25. M. Marcandier, *A Treatise on Hemp* (Boston, MA: 1766).

Nutritious, Healthy Hempseed

1. C. Sagan, *The Dragons of Eden* (London: H&J Publishing, 1977).

2. House Committee on Ways and Means, *National Institute of Oilseed Products Testimony to Congress. HR 6385*, April and May, 1937.

3. U. Erasmus, *Fats that Heal, Fats that Kill* (Burnaby, B.C.: Alive Books, 1993), 44.

4. N. Goundry, trans., *Da Ma*.

5. Furr, Marion, and Mahlberg, "Histochemical Analyses of Laticifers and Glandular Trichomes in *Cannabis sativa*," *Journal of Natural Products* 44 (1981): 153–59; Hemphill, Turner, and Mahlberg, "Cannabinoid Content of Individual Plant Organs from Different Geographical Strains of *C. sativa* L.," *Journal of Natural Products* 43 (1980): 112–22; G. M. Petwardhan, et al., "Gas-chromatographic Detection of Resins in Cannabis Seeds," *Indian Journal of Pharmaceutical Sciences* 40 (1978): 166–67.

6. Original Sources, Box 7137, Boulder, CO 80306.

7. L. Osburn, "Hempseed: The Most Nutritionally Complete Food in the World. Part 1," *Hemp Line Journal* 1 (1992): 14.

8. J. St. Angelo, et al., "Isolation of Edestin from Aleurone Grains of *Cannabis sativa,*" *Archives of Biochemistry and Biophysics* 124 (1968): 199–205.

9. Vichery, Smith, and Nolan, "A Substitute for Edestin," *Science* 92 (1940): 317–18.

10. L. Osburn, "Hempseed: The Most Nutritionally Complete Food in the World," 12, 14.

11. Erasmus, *Fats that Heal, Fats that Kill*, 127, 236–37, 285–291, 304.

12. Lees and Karel, *Omega-6 Essential Fatty Acids in Health and Disease.*

13. Adapted from K. Jones, *Nutritional and Medicinal Guide to Hemp Seed.* (Gibsons, B.C.: Rainforest Botanical Laboratory, 1995); D. F. Horrobin and M. S. Manku, *Omega-6 Essential Fatty Acids* (Alan R. Leis, 1990), 21–53.

14. A. Weil, "Therapeutic Hemp Oil," *Natural Health* (March/April, 1993): 10–12.

15. "If we were deprived of the use of hempseed, it would affect all the pigeon producers in the US, of which there are upwards of 40,000." R. G. Scarlett, of W.G. Scarlett Corp. of Baltimore, MD, House Committee on Ways and Means, *Transcript of the Hearing on HR 6385,* April and May, 1937.

16. J. D. Socias, *Cáñamo: El Maravilloso Mundo de las Hierbas* (Barcelona, Spain: Ed. Dalmau Socias, 1982, 1988).

17. Marcandier, *Treatise on Hemp*, 8–9.

Holistic Health and Hemp

1. B. Silver, "Deformed Frogs Alarm Students, Scientists," *San Francisco Examiner* (October 10, 1996).

2. G. A. Lower, "Flax and Hemp: From the Seed to the Loom," *Mechanical Engineering* (Feb. 26, 1937).

3. "Auto Body Made of Plastics Resists Denting under Hard Blows," *Popular Mechanics* (December 1941); "Car-maker Turns to Cannabis—for fibre," *Nature* 384 (1996): 95.

4. C. Conrad, *Hemp, Lifeline to the Future* (Los Angeles, CA: Creative Xpressions, 1994).

5. L. H. Dewey and J. L. Merrill, "Hemp Hurds as Paper-Making Material," *USDA Bulletin 404.* (Washington, D. C.: U.S. Govt. Printing Office, 1916).

6. House Committee on Ways and Means, *Transcript of the Hearing on HR 6385,* April and May, 1937.

7. FBN Director Harry Anslinger to Asst. Sec. Treasury Stephen B. Gibbons, Feb. 1, 1936, see D. F. Musto, *The American Disease: Origins of Narcotic Control* (Clinton, MA: Colonial Press Inc., 1973), 224.

8. *Yearbook of the U.S. Department of Agriculture, 1930* (Washington, DC: U.S. Government Printing Office, 1931).

9. Dewey, "Hemp," 305–326.

10. J. Herer, *Hemp and the Marijuana Conspiracy: The Emperor Wears No Clothes.* (Van Nuys, CA: HEMP Publishing, 1991).

11. "The mighty hemp plant enters as savior of the moor lands. It grows quick and large and helps cultivate the land.... It keeps the moor ground dark and healthy." *Die Lustige Hanffibel* (Berlin, Germany: Reich's Nutritional Institute, 1943).

12. T. W. Harvey, *USDA Extension Service Handbook on Agriculture and Home Economics* (Washington, DC: U.S. Government Printing Office, 1926), 616–17.

13. T. Morton, *New English Canaan* (1632), 64.

14. T. Paine, *Common Sense* (1776).

15. W. Brune, Soil Conservation Service. Testimony to the Senate Committee on Agriculture and Forestry (July 6, 1976); S. King, "Iowa Rain and Wind Deplete Farmlands," *New York Times* (Dececember 5, 1976), cited in *Vegetarian Times* (March 1985): 45–47.

16. USDA Soil Conservation Service. *Summary Report, 1987 National Resources Inventory. Statistical Bulletin 790,* December 1989.

17. F. M. Lappe, *Diet for a Small Planet* (New York: Ballantine Books, 1982), 80.

18. A. Barnum, "Many Mammal Species Described as Endangered," *San Francisco Chronicle* (October 4, 1996).

19. The 1930 drought had a good effect on hemp grown in Kentucky, Illinois, and Wisconsin. USDA, *The Official Record* (December 25, 1930): 3.

20. B. Goldman, *The Truth About Where You Live* (New York: Times Books, 1991); "Warning: Unsafe for Human Life," *Longevity* (August 1991): 22ff.

21. Cross, et al., "Current Issues in Food Production: A Perspective on Beef as a Component in Diets for Americans," *National Cattleman's Association* (April 1990): 526.

22. J. Cavender, cited in J. Phillips, "Authorities Examine Pot Claims," *Athens News* (November 16, 1989).

23. "EPA Study Reinforces Link between Dioxin and Cancer," *Buffalo News* (September 12, 1994).

24. "Hole in Ozone Layer Is Bigger than Ever, UN Official Says," *San Francisco Chronicle* (November 28, 1996).

25. Dewey, "Hemp," 305–26.

26. M. Hayes and H. Wilbur, Reports at National Research Council Conference (Irvine, CA: 1990); R. Cowen, "Vanishing Amphibians," *Science News* (1990).

27. Only 20% of the hurd was used to fuel the plant. Sackett and Hobbs, *Hemp: A War Crop* (New York: Mason and Hanger Co., 1942).

28. N. Strawn, "Alcohol Fuels: Alternatives for Today and the Future," *Biologue* (September 1990): 13–16.

29. D. Pimentel and M. Pimentel, *Food, Energy and Society* (1979), 59.
30. L. Brown of Worldwatch Institute. 1974 estimates, adjusted using 1988 figures from USDA *Agricultural Statistics, 1989.* Tables 74, High protein feeds, and 75, Feed concentrates fed to livestock & poultry; B. Resenberg, "Curb on US Waste Urged to Help the World's Hungry," *New York Times* (October 25, 1974); EarthSave, *Realities for the 90s* (Santa Cruz, CA: 1991).
31. I. Molotosky, "Animal Antibiotics Tied to Illness in Humans," *New York Times* (February 22, 1987).
32. P. Baraniecki, L. Grabowska, and J. Mankowski, *Biorohstoff Hanf* (Nova Inst., 1995).
33. A. Teramura, "University of Maryland Study," *Discover* (September 1989).
34. A. Haney and B. B. Kutscheid, "An Ecological Study of Naturalized Hemp (*Cannabis sativa* L.) in East-Central Illinois," *American Midland Naturalist* 93 (1975).
35. HIA, PO Box 1080, Occidental, CA 95456. (500) 442-4367 (500-HIA-Hemp).

The Age of Deceit

1. Quoted by Jack Anderson, *Washington Post* (June 24, 1972).
2. "Deglamorising cannabis," *Lancet* 346 (1995): 1241.
3. "Should the World Go to Pot?" *New Times* (February 7, 1991).
4. W. E. Dixon, "The Pharmacology of Cannabis indica," 1354–57.
5. Sallan, et al., "Antiemetics in Patients Receiving Chemotherapy for Cancer," 135; Vinciguerra, Moore, and Brennan, "Inhalation Marijuana as an Antiemetic for Cancer Chemotherapy," 525–27.
6. Doblin and Kleiman, "Marihuana as Anti-emetic Medicine: A Survey of Oncologists' Attitudes and Experiences," 1275–80.
7. "Scientists Unlocking Secrets of Marijuana's Effects," *Los Angeles Times* (December 6, 1996).
8. Soderstrom, et al., "Marijuana and alcohol use among 1023 trauma patients," *Archives of Survey* 123 (1988): 733–37.
9. H. Robbe and J. O'Hanlon, *HS 808 078: Marijuana and Actual Driving Performance* (Springfield, VA: US DOT Nat. Technical Information Service, 1993), 1.
10. "They kind of forget about the rest of the world. They're not intentionally cutting somebody off, [they're] just not seeing them." John Violanti, who helped conduct the study. "Sunday," *San Francisco Chronicle* (March 24, 1996).
11. A. Freco and L. Jenkins of the *London Times*, quoted in "Scientists Link Asthma, Cancer to Cell Phones," *San Francisco Examiner* (June 3, 1996).

12. D. Baum, *Smoke and Mirrors* (New York: Little, Brown and Co., 1996), 237, 240; A. Hoffman and J. Silvers, *Steal this Urine Test* (New York: Viking Press, 1987), 121, 123.

13. J. P. Morgan, "Marijuana Metabolism in the Context of Urine Testing," 107–15.

14. R. C. Kolodny, "Depression of Plasma Testosterone Levels after Chronic Intensive Marijuana Use," *NIDA Research Monograph Series No. 2* (1974): 30–31.

15. J. H. Mendelson, *New England Journal of Medicine* (November 1974).

16. G. Lean of the *London Independent*, quoted in "Low Sperm Counts May Be Due to Pesticides," *San Francisco Examiner* (June 30, 1996).

17. "Should the World Go to Pot?" 15.

18. "Teen Drug Use Highest in Study's History," *San Francisco Chronicle* (September 26, 1996); J. Brown, "Teenagers' Use of Drugs May Be Underestimated; Degree of Abuse Found to Be Far in Excess of Current Federal Estimates," *San Francisco Examiner* (September 26, 1996).

19. K. Fagan, "Just Say No groups Mark 10 Effective Years," *San Francisco Chronicle* (October 4, 1996).

20. L. Beil, "New Meaning for Chocolate High: Study Hints Sweet Is Similar to Marijuana," *San Francisco Examiner* (August 22, 1996); D. Piomelli, et. al., *Nature* (August 22, 1996).

The Legal Prognosis

1. T. Jefferson, "A Summary View of the Rights of British America (1774), in *Jefferson Writings*, M.D. Peterson, ed. (New York: The Library of America, 1984), 110.

2. *Report of the President's Advisory Commission on Narcotics and Drug Abuse* (1963).

3. P. Anderson, *High in America: The true story behind NORML and the politics of marijuana* (New York: Viking Press, 1981), 54.

4. Baum, *Smoke and Mirrors*, 9.

5. Speech at Anaheim, California (September 16, 1968).

6. Operations in Laos, under CIA operatives Theodore Shackley, Thomas Clines, and Richard Secord, were carried out by anticommunist Chinese Nationalists soldiers. A. McCoy, *The Politics of Heroin in Southeast Asia*.

7. Baum, *Smoke and Mirrors*, 54–55.

8. National Commission on Marihuana and Drug Abuse, *Marihuana: A Signal of Misunderstanding* (Washington, DC: U.S. Govt. Printing Office, 1972).

9. Constitution of the United States of America, Article VI.2.

10. Charter of the United Nations, Article 2.7.

11. Charter of the United Nations, Preamble.

12. Universal Declaration on Human Rights, Article 25.1.

13. Single Convention Treaty on Narcotic Drugs, Preamble, Article 28.

14. H. Anslinger, Testimony from Marijuana Tax Act Hearings (1937).

15. Sen. Robert LaFollette (1945).

16. The official hempseed sample of the United States is kept at the USDA Seed Bank in Colorado Springs, CO. DEA form 225 and a permit are required to possess fertile seed here.

17. F. Young, DEA Chief Administrative Law Judge, *In the Matter of Marijuana Rescheduling Petition* , Docket No. 86-22. (Washington, DC: September 6, 1988).

18. Silberman, Buckley, and Henderson, Circuit Judges, *In the Matter of Marijuana Rescheduling Petition* , Ninth circuit court of appeals (April 1991).

19. National Association of Attorneys General, *Therapeutic use of marijuana*, Committee on Criminal Law and Law Enforcement XI (June 25, 1983).

20. *U.S. v. Randall*, 104 Wash. DC Superior Court (1976), Daily Law rep. 2249; *Florida v. Musikka*, No. 88-4395 CFA, 17th Judicial Circuit Court (December 28, 1988).

21. S. Hadly, "Ex-Moorpark Official gets probation," *Los Angeles Times* (July 4, 1996).

22. T. Mauro, "Legalize Marijuana, Prominent Jurist Says," *USA Today* (September 14, 1995).

23. "State Should be Allowed to Study Medical Pot Use," *Seattle Times* (December 13, 1996).

24. "Government Extinguishes Marijuana Access, Advocates Smell Politics," *JAMA* 267 (May 20, 1992): 2573.

25. "Pall of Turmoil and Concern Over Medical Marijuana Law: Good Judgment of Doctors is Only Real Protection for Now," *Los Angeles Times* (November 10, 1996).

26. Signed ballot arguments, *California Ballot Pamphlet* (August 12, 1996): 60–61.

27. *San Francisco Chronicle* (September 28, 1996).

28. *San Francisco Chronicle* (November 10, 1996).

29. G. Martin, "Both Sides Say 215 Decriminalizes Pot Use," *San Francisco Chronicle* (November 7, 1996).

30. "Pall of Turmoil and Concern Over Medical Marijuana Law: Good Judgment of Doctors is the Only Real Protection for Now," *Los Angeles Times* (November 10, 1996).

31. *Los Angeles Times* (December 16, 1996).

32. R. Salladay, "Lungren Lays Down Medical Pot Law," *Oakland Tribune* (December 4, 1996).

33. AMA, *Code of Medical Ethics*, 2.17 (1994).

34. "Scientists Advocate Marijuana for the Ill," *Reuter* (November 15, 1994).

35. R. Doblin, "AIDS Wasting Syndrome Protocol Update," *MAPS Bulletin* (Summer 1996): 67.
36. E. Larson, A.J. Ellsworth, and J. Oas, "Randomized Clinical Trials in Single Patients During a 2-Year Period," *Journal of the American Medical Association* 270 (December 8, 1993): 2708–2712.
37. D. Spyker, CDER Research Proposal RFP: Multicenter single-patient randomized clinical trials of Δ-9-THC (Submitted February 12, 1991).
38. C. Lochhead, "Lungren in Washington for Briefing on Pot Law," *San Francisco Chronicle* (December 14, 1996).
39. G. Martin, "Prop 215 Attacked in US Senate," *San Francisco Chronicle* (December 3, 1996).
40. "Governor Ponders Vetoes of 200, 201," *Arizona Republic* (November 6, 1996).
41. Marijuana Policy Project, *How Can a State Legislature Enable Patients to Use Medicinal Marijuana Despite Federal Prohibition*, PO Box 77492, Washington, DC, 20013. 202-462-5747. Internet: http://www.mpp.org.
42. Washington Post Service, "Night Goggles Illuminate Military's Drug Role," *Oakland Tribune* (November 30, 1996).

Appendix A

1. Clarke and Pate, "Medical Marijuana," 9–12.
2. F. L. Young, DEA Chief Adminstrative Law Judge, *In the Matter of Marijuana Rescheduling Petition*, Docket No 86-22 (Washington, DC: Sept. 6, 1988).

Bibliography

Abel, Ernest L., *Marihuana: The First 12,000 Years* (Plenum Press, New York, NY), 1980.

Adams, Roger, Marijuana. *Science* 92:115–118.

Adler M. W., & Geller, E.B., Ocular effects of cannabinoids. In *Cannabinoids as Therapeutic Agents*, R. Mechoulam, Ed. (CRC Press, Boca Raton, FL), pp. 51–70, 1986.

Aldrich, Michael, *High Times Encyclopedia* (Trans High Publishing, New York, NY), p. 118, 1978.

Allentuck, S., & Bowman, K. M., The psychiatric aspects of marihuana intoxication. *American Journal of Psychiatry* 99:248–251 (1942).

Alliance for Cannabis Therapeutics, No accepted medical value? *ACT News* Spring (1995).

American Medical Association, *Code of Medical Ethics*, 2.17, 1994.

American Public Health Association, Resolution No. 7014: Marijuana and the law. *APHA Public Policy Statements* (APHA, Washington, DC), 1948–present, cumulative.

Ames, F., A clinical and metabolic study of acute intoxication with *Cannabis sativa* and its role in the model psychoses. *Journal of Mental Sciences* 104(437): 972–999 (1958).

Anandakanda, 10th C. Trans., p. 236, 1952.

Anderson, Jack, *Washington Post* 24:31 (June 1972).

Anderson, Patrick, *High in America: The True Story behind NORML and the Politics of Marijuana* (Viking Press, New York, NY), p. 54, 1981.

Anicia Juliana, 512.

Anslinger, H. J., *Testimony from Marijuana Tax Act Hearings*, 1937.

Associated Press, Court to rule on immunity for private prison guards. *San Francisco Chronicle* Nov. 28:A-20 (1996).

Associated Press, KY troopers kill man defending his pot plants. *Arizona Daily Sun* Aug. 10 (1993).

Associated Press, Surgeon general nominee backs use of marijuana as medicine. *Los Angeles Times* Dec. 20:A-27 (1920).

Associated Press, Teen drug use highest in study's history. *San Francisco Chronicle* Sept. 26:A-4 (1996).

Arkansas v. Tom Brown, 1995.

Atharva Veda, viii. 8.3; xi. 8(6).15.

Auto body made of plastics resists denting under hard blows. *Popular Mechanics* December (1941).

Ball, M.V., Effects of haschisch not due to cannabis indica. *Therapeutic Gazette* 34:777–780 (1910).

Baraniecki, P, Grabowska, L., & Mankowski, J., *Biorohstoff Hanf* (Institute of Natural Fibers, Nova Institute, Poznan, Poland), 1995.

Barnum, Alex, Many mammal species described as endangered. *San Francisco Chronicle* Oct. 4:A-1 (1996).

Batho, Dr. R., Cannabis indica. *British Medical Journal* May 26:1002 (1883).

Baum, Dan, *Smoke and Mirrors.* (Little, Brown), pp. 237, 240.

Bazzaz, Dusek, Seigler, & Haney, *Photosynthesis and Cannabinoid Content of Temperate and Tropical Populations of Cannabis* (University of Illinois Press, Urbana, IL), October 1974.

Beil, L., New meaning for chocolate high: Study hints sweet is similar to marijuana. *San Francisco Examiner* Aug. 22:A-12 (1996).

Bell, S. J., *Positive Nutrition for HIV Infection and AIDS* (Chronimed Publishing), 1996.

Bellavite, Paolo, & Signorini, Andrea, *Homeopathy: A Frontier in Medical Science.*

Benet, S., Early diffusion and folk uses of hemp. In *Cannabis and Culture,* V. Rubin, Ed. (Mouton, The Hague, Netherlands), 1975.

Bennet, Chris, Osburn, Lynn, & Judy, *Green Gold the Tree of Life, Marijuana in Magic and Religion* (Access Unlimited, Frazier Park, CA), pp. 102, 104, 105, 108, 144, 1995.

Berger J., Mother's homemade marijuana: A plan to aid her son leads to arrest and push for change. *NY Times* Oct. 11 (1993).

Beringer, K., et al., Zur klinik des hashischrauschec. *Der Nervenarzt.* 5:337–350 (1932).

Beutler, John A., & Der Marderosian, Ara H., Chemotaxonomy of cannabis. I. Cross-breeding between *Cannabis sativa* and *C. ruderalis,* with analysis of cannabinoid content. *Economic Botany* 32(4):387–394 (1978).

Bhagavat-purana, Canto 5, Chap. 24, p. 16.

Biernson, G., Data on storage of marijuana in the body. *Drug Awareness Information Newsletter* March (1988).

Birch, E. C., The use of Indian hemp in the treatment of chronic chloral and chronic opium poisoning. *Lancet* 1:624 (1889).

Boericke, William, Comprising the characteristic and guiding symptoms of the remedies. *Homeopathic Materia Medica* (Woolnough Book Binding Ltd., Northamptonshire, UK), pp. 160–162, 1987.

Bonnie, R. J., & Whitebread, C. H., *The Marijuana Conviction: A History of Marijuana Prohibition in the United States* (University Press of Virginia, Charlottesville, VA), 1974.

Booth, W., Marijuana receptor exists in brain, study confirms. *Washington Post* Aug. 9 (1990).

Brazil, E., Drug czar takes aim at pot law. *San Francisco Examiner* Dec. 23:A-1 (1996).

Brecher, Edward M., & Editors of Consumer Reports, *Licit and Illicit Drugs. The Consumers Union Report* (Little Brown & Co.), pp. 397–398, 1972.

Brill, Crumpton, Frank, Hochman, Lomax, McGlothlin, & West, The marijuana problems [UCLA Interdepartmental Conference]. *Annals of Internal Medicine* 73(3): 449–465 (1970).

British Pharmacopoeia C., 1949. Cited in *Martindale, The Extra Pharmacopoeia* (The Pharmaceutical Press, London), 26 ed., p. 377, 1972.

Brown, J., Teenagers' use of drugs may be underestimated: Degree of abuse found to be far in excess of current federal estimates. *San Francisco Examiner* Sept. 26:A-2 (1996).

Brown, Dr. John, *Cannabis indica*: A valuable remedy in menorrhagia. *British Medical Journal* 1:1002 (1883).

Brune, William, *Testimony to U.S. Senate Committee on Agriculture and Forestry* (Soil Conservation Service, Des Moines, IA), July 6, 1976.

Caldwell, D. F., Myers, S. A., & Domino, E. F., Effects of marihuana smoking on sensory thresholds in man. In *Psychotomimetic Drugs*, D. Efron, Ed. (Raven Press, New York), pp. 299–321, 1970.

Caldwell, Myers, Domino, & Merriam, Auditory and visual threshold effects of marihuana in man. *Perceptual and Motor Skills* 29:755–759 (1969); Addendum. *Perceptual and Motor Skills* 29:922 (1969).

California Ballot Pamphlet, Certified by Secretary of State Bill Jones, pp. 60–61, Aug. 12, 1996.

Cannabis clubs open for medicinal business. *USA Today* Oct. 1:B-1, B-5 (1993).

Car-maker turns to cannabis—for fibre. *Nature* 384:95 (1996).

Caraka samhita, Sutra 1:15.

Carlini, E. A., & Cunha, J. A., Hypnotic and anti-epileptic effects of CBD. *Journal of Clinical Pharmacology* 21:417S–427S (1981).

Carlini, Masur, et al., Possivel Efeito Hipnotico do CBD no ser Humano. *Ciencia E Cultura* 31(3):315–322 (1979) [in Portuguese].

Carter, V.G., & Dale, T., *Topsoil and Civilization* (University of Oklahoma Press, Norman, OK), 1974.

Case Histories, *Human Rights 95: Atrocities of the Drug War* (Oakland, CA).

Cavender, Jim, Authorities examine pot claims. *Athens News* [Athens, OH] 13:92 (Nov. 16, 1989).

Chait, L. D., Δ-9-THC content and human marijuana self-administration (Pritzker School of Medicine, University of Chicago, IL), 1989.

Cherniak, Laurence, *The Great Books of Hashish* (Kulu Trading), 1995.

Chopra, I. C., & Chopra, R. N., The use of the cannabis drugs in India. *UN Bulletin on Narcotics* 9(1):4–29 (1957).

Clark, L. D. Hughes, R., & Nakashima, E. N., Behavioral effects of marihuana: Experimental studies. *Archives of General Psychiatry* 23:193–195 (1970).

Clark, L. D., & Nakashima, E. N., Experimental studies of marihuana. *American Journal of Psychiatry* 125:379–384 (1968).

Clark, L. D., Hughes R., & Nakashima, E. N., Behavioral effects of marihuana: Experimental studies. *Archives of General Psychiatry* 23:193–198 (1970).

Clarke, R. C., & Pate, D. W., Medical marijuana. *Journal of the International Hemp Association* 1:9–12 (1994).

Clayman, Charles B., Ed., *The American Medical Association Encyclopedia of Medicine* (Random House, New York), 1989.

Clifford D. B., THC for tremor in multiple sclerosis. *Annals of Neurology* 13:669–671 (1983).

Cockburn, L., *Out of Control* (Atlantic Monthly Press, New York), 1987.

Cognition and long term use of ganga. *Science* 213:465–466 (1981).

Cohen, Dr. Sidney, & Stillman, Richard, Eds., *Therapeutic Potential of Marijuana* (Plenum Press, New York), 1976.

Cohen, Dr. Sidney, Marijuana as medicine. *Psychology Today* April:60 (1978).

Cohen, Dr. Sidney, Therapeutic aspects. *Marihuana* (NIDA monograph, Washington, DC), Chap. 9, pp. 194–225, 1976.

Cohen, Dr. Sidney, *Therapeutic Potential of Marijuana's Components* (American Council on Marijuana and Other Psychoactive Drugs), 1982.

Colasanti, B. K., Review: Ocular hypotensive effect of marihuana carmabinoids: Correlate of central action on separate phenomenon. *Journal of Ocular Pharmacology* 2(3):295–304 (1986).

Cone, Johnson, Paul, Mell, & Mitchell, Marijuana-laced brownies: Behavioral effects, physiologic effects and urinalysis. *Journal of Analytical Toxicology* 12(4):169–175 (1988).

Cone, Welch, & Lange, Clonidine partially blocks the physiologic effects but not the subjective effects produced by smoking marijuana. *Pharmacology, Biochemistry and Behavior* 29(3):649–652 (1988).

Conrad, Chris, *Hemp, Lifeline to the Future* (Creative Xpressions, Los Angeles, CA), 1993, 1994.

Consroe, et al., Open label evaluation of cannabidiol in dystonic movement disorders. *International Journal of Neuroscience* 30:277–282 (1986).

Constitution of the United States of America, Article VI.2.

Conti, Johannesen, Musty, & Consroe, Anti-dyskinetic effects of cannabidiol. *Proceedings of the International Congress on Marijuana, Melbourne, Australia,* 1987.

Controlled Substances Act of 1970, Pub. L. 91-513. October 27, 1970. 21 USC 801 et. seq.

Cooley, Donald, Ed., *After-40 Health and Medical Guide* (Better Homes &

Gardens), p. 24, 1980.

Cowen, R., Vanishing amphibians. *Science News* (1990).

Coy, Waller, Chemistry of marijuana. *Pharmacological Reviews* 23:4 (1971).

Crancer, Dille, Delay, Wallace, & Haykin, Simulated driving performance. *Science* 164:851–854 (1969).

Cross, Byers, et al., A perspective on beef as a component in diets for Americans. *Minutes of National Cattleman's Association* April:526 (1990).

Culpeper, N., *Complete Herbal* (Richard Evans Co., London), p. 91, 1814.

Cunha, Carlini, Pereira, et al., Chronic administration of cannabidiol to healthy volunteers and epileptic patients. *Pharmacology* 21:175–185 (1980).

Dalman, Jose, Ed., Cáñamo. *El Maravilloso Mundo de las Hierbas* (Dalman Socias, Barcelona, Spain), 1988.

DaOrta, Garcia, *Colloquies on the Simples and Drugs of India* (Henry Southern, London), 1913 [original 1563].

Dash, Bhagwan Yaidya, Ex-deputy adviser (Ayurveda) Ministry of Health and Family Welfare, *Fundamentals of Ayurvedic Medicine* (Bansal & Co., New Delhi, India), pp. ix–xvi, 141–157, 1984.

Dash, Bhagwan, *The Yoga of Herbs,* pp. 107–110.

Davis, J. A., & Ramsey, H. H., Anti-epileptic action of marihuana-active substances. *Federation Proceedings* 8:284–285 (1949).

de Meijer, E. P. M., Characterization of Cannabis accessions with regard to cannabinoid content in relation to other plant characters. *Euphytica* 62:187–200 (1992).

de Meijer, E. P. M., Hemp variations as pulp source researched in The Netherlands. *Pulp and Paper* July:41–43 (1993).

Dewey, L. H., & Merrill, J. L., Hemp hurds as paper-making material. *USDA Bulletin* (U.S. Govt. Printing Office, Washington, DC), No. 404, 1916.

Dewey, Lyster H. [Chief botanist, fiber plant specialist, USDA], Hemp. *Yearbook of the United States Department of Agriculture, 1913* (Government Printing Office, Washington, DC), 1914.

Diamond, Harvey & Marilyn, *Fit for Life* (Warner Books, New York), 1987.

Die Lustige Hanffibel (Reich's Nutritional Institute, Berlin), 1943.

Dioscorides, *Materia Medica.* 3.165, 70 A.D.

Dixon, Walter Ernest, The pharmacology of *Cannabis indica. British Medical Journal* Nov. 11:1354–1357 (1897).

Doblin, R., & Kleiman, M., Marihuana as anti-emetic medicine: A survey of oncologists' attitudes and experiences. *Journal of Clinical Oncology* July:1275–1280 (1991).

Doblin, Rick, AIDS wasting syndrome protocol update. *MAPS Bulletin* [Multidisciplinary Association for Psychedelic Studies] 4(3):67 (Summer 1996).

Domino, E. F., Human pharmacology of marihuana smoking [Minutes of American Society for Clinical Pharmacology and Therapeutics, 1970]. *Journal of Clinical Pharmacology Therapeutics* (1971).

Douglas, J., On the use of Indian hemp in Chorea. *Edinburgh Medical Journal* 14:777–784 (1883).

Du Pont, Lammont, President of Du Pont. From test tube to you. *Popular Mechanics* June:805 (1939).

Du Pont, Lammont, *Annual Report* (1937).

Dwarakanath, S. C., Use of opium and cannabis in the traditional systems of medicine in India. *UN Bulletin on Narcotics* 17(1):15–19 (1965).

EarthSave, *Realities for the 90s* (Santa Cruz, CA), 1991.

Edes, R. T., Cannabis indica. *Boston Medical Surgery Journal* Sept. 14:129–273 (1893).

Edinburgh New Dispensatory (W. Creech Co., Edinburgh, Scotland), p. 126, 1794.

Editorial: Deglamorising cannabis. *Lancet* 346(8985):1241 (1995).

Editorial: State shuld be allowed to study medical pot use. *Seattle Times* Dec. 13:B-6 (1996).

Effects of cannabis and alcohol during labour. *Journal of the American Medical Association* 94:1165 (1930).

El Cáñamo, *El Mundo Marvilloso de las Hierbas* (Barcelona, Spain).

El-Mallakh, R. S., *Marijuana and Migraine* (University of California Health Center, Neurology Department, Farmington, CT), 1987.

Elias, M., Study says cigarettes cut down on virility. *Courier News* May 16:A-11 (1991).

ElSolhy, M. A., et al., Constituents of *Cannabis sativa* L. XXIV: The potency of confiscated marijuana, hashish and hash oil over a 10-year period. *Journal of Forensic Sciences* 29 (1984).

ElSolhy, M. A., et al., *Report on the Potency of Confiscated Marijuana* (University of Mississippi), 1993.

Erasmus, Udo, *Fats That Heal, Fats That Kill* (Alive Books, Burnaby, British Columbia, Canada), p. 44, 1993.

Evans, Fred J., Cannabinoids: The separation of central from peripheral effects on a structural basis. *Planta Medica* 57(1): S60(1991).

Ewald, E. B., *Recipes for a Small Planet* (Ballantine Books, New York), 1973.

Fagan, K., Just Say No groups mark 10 effective years. *San Franciso Chronicle* Oct. 4:A-21 (1996).

Feeney, D., Marijuana use among epileptics. *Journal of the American Medical Association* 235:1105(1976).

Ferenczy, L., Gracza, L., & Jakobey, I., An antibacterial preparation from hemp (*Cannabis sativa*, L.). *Naturwissenschaften* 45:188 (1958).

Fink, M., The biology of cannabis: The state of our knowledge, 1970. Paper presented at American Public Health Symposium on Cannabis, San Francisco, May 13, 1970.

Fischlowitz, G. G., Poisoning by Cannabis indica. *Medical Record* 50:280–281(1896).

Florida v. Musikka. No. 88-4395 CFA, 17th Judicial Circuit Court, Dec. 28, 1988.

Flowers, Tom, *Marijuana Herbal Cookbook* (Flowers Publishing, Berkeley, CA), 1995.

Foltin, Capriotti, et al., Effects of marijuana, cocaine and task performance on cardiovascular responsivity. *NIDA Monograph* June 16–18:259–265 (1986).

Foltin, R. W, Fischman, M. W., & Byrne, M. F., Effects of smoked marijuana on food intake and body weight of humans living in a residential laboratory. *Appetite* 11:1–14 (1988).

Foltz, Kinzer, Mitchell, & Truitt, The fate of cannabinoid components of marihuana during smoking. *Journal of Analytical Chemistry* (1971).

Formukong, Evans, & Evans, Analgesic and anti-inflammatory activity of constituents of *Cannabis sativa* L. *Inflammation* 12(4):361–371 (1988).

Fournier and Paris, Paper-making type of hemp (*Cannabis sativa*, L.) cultivated in France: Constituents compared to those of marijuana. *Plantes Medicinales et Phytotherapie* 13(2):116–121 (1979) [in French].

Fournier, Gilbert, et al., Identification of a new chemotype in *Cannabis sativa*: Cannabigerol dominant plants, biogenetic and agronomic prospects. *Planta Medica* 53(3):277–280 (1987).

Fox, R. E., Headaches, a study of some common forms, with especial reference to arterial tension and to treatment. *Lancet* 3:307–309 (1897).

Frank, Hepler, Stier, & Rickles, Marihuana, tobacco and functions affecting driving. In *Minutes of American Psychiatric Association Annual Meeting* (Washington, DC), May 1971.

Fraser, J., Treatment of tetanus with Cannabis indica. *Medical Times Gazette* Feb. 7:1 (1862).

Freco, Adam, & Jenkins, Lin, Scientists link asthma, cancer to cell phones. *San Francisco Examiner* June 3:A-2 (1996).

Fried, P. A., Postnatal consequences of maternal marijuana use. *NIDA Monograph Series* 113:61–72 (1985).

Fuchs, Leonhart, *De Historia Stirpium* (Basel), 1542.

Furr, Marion, & Mahlberg, Paul G., Histochemical analyses of laticifers and glandular trichomes in *Cannabis sativa*. *Journal of Natural Products* 44(2):153–159 (1981).

Galen, Claudius, *De Facultatibus Alimentorum*, 100.49.

Gary, N. E., & Keylon, V., Intravenous administration of marihuana. *Journal of the American Medical Association* 11(3):501 (1970).

Goldman, B., *The Truth About Where You Live* (Times Books, New York), 1991.

Goundry, Norman, translator, *Da Ma (Hemp. Marijuana — Cannabis sativa)*, Translations from the Ben Cao Gang Mu (Madeira Park, British Columbia, Canada), 1995.

Government extinguishes marijuana access, advocates smell politics. *Journal of the American Medical Association* 267(19):2573 (1992).

Governor ponders vetoes of 200, 201. *AZ Republic* Nov. 6:1 (1996).

Graham, J. D. P., The bronchodilator action of cannabinoids. In *Cannabinoids as Therapeutic Agents*, R. Mechoulam, Ed. (CRC Press, Boca Raton, FL), pp. 147–158, 1986.

Green, K., & McDonald, T. F., Ocular toxicology of marijuana: Update. *Journal of Toxicology* 6(4):239–382 (1987).

Grinspoon, L., & Bakalar, J. B., Commentary: Marihuana as medicine: A plea for reconsideration. *Journal of the American Medical Association* 273(23):1875–1876 (1995).

Grinspoon, L., & Bakalar, J. B., *Marijuana, The Forbidden Medicine* (Yale University Press, New Haven, CT), 1993.

Hadly, Scott, Ex-Moorpark Official gets probation. *Los Angeles Times* July 4 (1996).

Haney, Alan, & Kutscheid, B. B., An ecological study of naturalized hemp (*Cannabis sativa*, L.) in East-Central Illinois. *American Midland Naturalist* 93:1 (1975).

Hare, Hobart Amory, *Practical Therapeutics* (Philadelphia, PA), p. 181, 1922.

Harris, L. S., Munson, A. E., & Carchman, R. A., Antitumor properties of cannabinoids. In *The Pharmacology of Marihuana*, M. C. Braude and S. Szara, Eds. (Raven, New York), pp. 773–776, 1976.

Harvey, T. W., *USDA Extension Service Handbook on Agriculture and Home Economics* (Washington, DC), pp. 616–617, October 1926.

Hayes, Marc, & Wilbur, Henry, *Biologist Reports* (National Research Council Conference, Irvine, CA), 1990.

Hemenway, S., Poisoning by strychnine, successfully treated by cannabis. *Pacific Medicine and Surgery Journal* 10:113–114 (1867).

Hemp, *Encyclopaedia Britannica* (London), 1957.

Hemphill, Turner, & Mahlberg, Cannabinoid content of individual plant organs from different geographical strains of *C. sativa* L. *Journal of Natural Products* 43(1):112–122 (1980).

Hepler, R., & Petrus, R., Experiences with administration of marijuana to glaucoma patients. In *The Pharmacology of Marihuana*, M. C. Braude and S. Szara, Eds. (Raven Press, New York), pp. 63–94, 1976.

Hepler, R. S., & Frank, I. M., Marihuana smoking and intraocular pressure. *Journal of the American Medical Association* 217:1392 (1971).

Hepler, R. S., Frank I. M., & Ungerleider, J. T., The effects of marijuana smoking on pupillary size. *American Journal of Opthalmology* (1971).

Herer, Jack, *Hemp and the Marijuana Conspiracy: The Emperor Wears No Clothes* (HEMP Publishing, Van Nuys, CA), p. 39, 1991.

Herodotus, *Histories IV, 450 BC* (University Press, Cambridge, MA), pp. 74–76, 1906.

Himmelsbach, C. K., Treatment of the morphine abstinence syndrome with a synthetic cannabis-like compound. *Southern Medical Journal* 37:26–29 (1944).

Hine, Friedman, Torrelio, & Gershon, Blockage of morphine abstinence by Δ-9-THC. *Science* 190:590–591 (1975).

Hoffman, Abbie, & Silvers, Jonathan, *Steal This Urine Test* (Penguin Books/ Viking Press, New York), pp. 121, 123, 1987.

Holding, R., Legal experts charge conflict in prison probe. *San Francisco Chronicle* Dec. 23:A-1 (1996).

Hollister, L. E., Hunger and appetite after single doses of marihuana, ethanol and dextroamphetamine. *Clinical Pharmacology and Therapeutics* (1972).

Hollister, L. E., Man and marijuana. *Science* 172:21–29 (1971).

Hollister, L. E., Steroids and moods: Correlations in schizophrenics and subjects treated with LSD, mescaline, THC, and synhexyl. *Journal of Clinical Pharmacology* 9:24–29 (1969).

Hollister, L. E., & Gillespie, H. K., Marihuana, ethanol and dextroamphetamine: Mood and mental function alterations. *Archives of General Psychiatry* 23:199–203 (1970).

Hollister, L. E., & Moore, F., Urinary catecholamine excretion following LSD in man. *Psychopharmacologia (Berlin)* 11:270 (1967).

Hollister, L. E., & Moore, F., Urinary catecholamine excretion following mescaline in man. *Biochemistry Pharmacology* 17:2015 (1968).

Hollister, L. E., Richards, R. K., & Gillespie, H. K., Comparison of THC and synhexyl in man. *Clinical Pharmacology and Therapeutics* 9:783–791 (1968).

Hollister, L. E., Sherwood, S. L., & Cavasino, A., Marihuana and the human electroencephalogram. *Pharmacological Research Communications* (1971).

Holy Bible, Genesis 1:29; Ezekiel 34:29; Revelation 11:18, 22:1–2.

Horrobin, D. F., & Manku, M. S., *Omega-6 Essential Fatty Acids* (Alan R. Leis), pp. 21–53, 1990.

Institute of Medicine, *Marijuana and Health* (National Academy Press, Washington, DC), 1982.

Isbell, Gorodetsky, Jasinski, Claussen, Von Spulek, & Korte, Effects of Δ-9-trans-THC in man. *Psychopharmacologia (Berlin)* 11:184–188 (1967).

Isbell, H., & Jasinski, D. R., A comparison of LSD-25 with Δ-9-THC and attempted cross tolerance between LSD and THC. *Psychopharmacologia* 14:115–123 (1969).

Isbell, Jasinski, Gorodetsky, Korte, Claussen, Haage, Sieper, & Von Spulak, Studies on THC. *Bulletin, Problems of Drug Dependence* [Minutes of 29th meeting, Lexington, KY, Feb. 13–16, 1967] (National Academy of Sciences, Division Medical Science, Washington, DC), pp. 4832–4846, 1967.

Jahr, G. H. G., *New Homeopathic Pharmacopoeia and Posology of the Preparation of Homeopathic Medicines* (J. Dobson, Philadelphia, PA), p. 137, 1842.

Jefferson, Thomas, A summary view of the rights of British America, 1774. In *Jefferson Writings*, Peterson, Ed. (The Library of America, New York), p. 110, 1984.

Johnson, Melvin, Althius, et al., Selective and potent analgesics derived from cannabinoids. *Journal of Clinical Pharmacology* 21:271S–282S (1981).

Jones, Kenneth, *Nutritional and Medicinal Guide to Hemp Seed* (Rainforest Botanical Laboratory, Gibsons, British Columbia, Canada), 1995.

Jones, R., & Stone, G., Psychological studies of marijuana and alcohol in man. *Psychopharmacologia (Berlin)* 18:108–117 (1970).

Jubácek, J., A contribution to the treatment of sinusitis maxillaris (Czechoslavakia). *Acta Univ. Palack. Olomuc.*, 207 (1961).

Jubácek, J., A study of the effect of c. indica in otorhinolaryngology (Czechoslavakia). *Acta Univ. Palack. Olomuc.*, 83 (1955).

Kabelik, J., Krejci, Z., & Santavy, F., Cannabis as a medicament. *UN Bulletin on Narcotics* 12(3):5–23 (1960).

Kambui, Somayah, Editorial. *Crescent Star News* (Crescent Alliance Sickle Cell Self Help Group, Los Angeles), 1992.

Karler, R., & Turkanis, S. A., The cannabinoids as potential anti-epileptics. *Journal Clinical Pharmacology* 21:437S–448S (1981).

Karniol, I. G., & Carlini, E. A., Pharmacological interaction between cannabidiol and Δ 9-THC. *Psychopharmacologia* 33:53–70 (1973).

Karniol, I. G., Shirakawa, I., et al., Cannabidiol interferes with the effects of Δ-9-THC in man. *European Journal of Pharmacy* 28:172–177 (1974).

Kemmoku, A., et al., Effect of *Cannabis sativa* seed oil on the serum cholesterol level in the rats fed on high cholesterol diet. *Bulletin of the Faculty of Education, Utsonomiya University*, 42(2):165–172 (1992) [in Japanese].

King, S., Iowa rain and wind deplete farmlands. *New York Times* Dec. 5:61 (1976).

Kleijnen, J., Knipschild, P., & ter Riet, Gerben, Clinical trials of homeopathy. *British Medical Journal* 302(6772):316–318 (1991).

Kolodny, R. C. [Masters and Johnson Sex Research Center, St. Louis, MO], Depression of plasma testosterone levels after chronic intensive marijuana use. *NIDA Research Monograph Series 2* Nov.:30–31 (1974).

Kotin, Post, & Goodwin, Delta-9 THC in depressed patients. *Archives of General Psychiatry* 28:345–348 (1973).

Krejci, Z., On the problem of substances with antibacterial action: Cannabis effect. *Casopis Lekaru Ceskych* 43:1351–1354 (1961).

Lamarck, Jean, *Encyclopedia*, Vol. 1, p. 695, 1788.

Lancz, Specter, & Brown, Suppressive effect of Δ-9-THC on herpes simplex virus infectivity in vitro. *Proceedings of the Society for Experimental Biology and Medicine* 196:401–404 (1991).

Lancz, Specter, Brown, Hackney, & Friedman, Interaction of Δ-9-THC with herpes viruses and cultural conditions associated with drug-induced anti-cellular effects. In *Drugs of Abuse, Immunity and Imunodeficiency*, Friedman, et al., Eds. (Plenum Press, New York), pp. 287–304, 1991.

Lansky, Philip S., Marijuana as medicine? *Health World* February:46–49

(1991).

Lappe, F. M., *Diet for a Small Planet* (Ballantine Books, New York), p. 80, 1982.

Larson, E. B., Ellsworth, A. J., & Oas, Janet, Randomized clinical trials in single patients during a 2-year period. *Journal of the American Medical Association* 270(22):2708–2712 (1993.

Latta, R. P., & Eaton, B. J., Seasonal fluctuations in Cannabinoid content of Kansas marijuana. *Economic Botany* 29:153–163 (1975).

Lean, Geoffrey, *London Independent.* Low sperm counts may be due to pesticides. *San Francisco Examiner* June 30:A-11 (1996).

Lees, R. S., & Karel, M., Eds., *Omega-6 Essential Fatty Acids in Health and Disease* (Dekker, New York), 1990.

Leger, C., & Nahas, G., Kinetics of cannabinoid distribution and storage with special reference to brain and testes. *Journal of Clinical Pharmacology* August (1981).

Lemberger, Silberstein, Axelrod, & Kopin, Marihuana: Studies on the disposition and metabolism of Δ-9-THC in man. *Science* 170:1320–1322 (1970).

Lerner, M., Marihuana: THC and related compounds. *Science* 140:175–176 (1963).

Lerner, M., Mills, A. L., & Mount, S. F., *Journal of Forensic Science* 8:126 (1963).

Leveritt, M., Reefer Madness: While courts send users to prison, scientists find little to support dangers of pot. *Arkansas Times* Sept. 16:11 (1993).

Lindemann, E., The neuro-physiological effects of intoxicating drugs. *American Journal of Psychiatry* 90:1007–1037 (1933–1934).

Lochhead, C., Lungren in Washington for briefing on pot law. *San Francisco Chronicle* Dec. 14:A-7 (1996).

Loewe, S., & Goodman, L. S., Anti-convulsant action of marihuana-active substances. *Federation Proceedings* 6(1):352 (1947).

Loewe, S., The active principles of cannabis and the pharmacology of the cannabinols. *Arch. Exper. Path. u Pharmakol.* 211:175–193 (1950) [in German].

Lower, George A., Flax and hemp: From the seed to the loom. *Mechanical Engineering* Feb. 26 (1937).

Loziers, Ralph [National Institute of Oilseed Products], *Transcript of the Hearing on HR 6385*, Committee on Ways and Means, House of Representatives, 75c 1s. April 27–30, May 4, 1937.

Mahabharata, I 76. 43–68.

Malec, Harvey, & Cayner, Cannabis' effect on spasticity in spinal cord injury. *Archives of Physical and Medical Rehabilitation* 35:198 (1982).

Mann, P. E. G., Finley, T. N., & Ladman, A. J., Marihuana smoking: A study of its effects on alveolar lining material and pulmonary macrophages recovered by bronchopulmonary lavage. *Journal of Clinical Investigations* June:60a–61a (1970).

Manno, J. E., Clinical investigations with marihuana and alcohol, (Department of Pharmacology and Toxicology, Indiana University), Doctoral thesus, 1970.

Manno, Kiplinger, Bennett, Hanna, & Forney, Comparative effects of smoking marihuana and motor and mental performance in humans. *Clinical Pharmacology and Therapeutics* 11(6):808–815 (1970).

Marcandier, M., *A Treatise on Hemp* (Boston, MA), 1766.

Marihuana and Health, A report to Congress from the Secretary (U.S. Department of Health, Education and Welfare), Section III, March 1971.

Marijuana may aid night vision. *Los Angeles Times* July 1:B-3 (1991).

Martin, G., Both sides say 215 decriminalizes pot use. *San Francisco Chronicle* Nov. 7:A-17 (1996).

Martin, G., Prop 215 attacked in U.S. Senate. *San Francisco Chronicle* Dec. 3:A-1 (1996).

Martindale, *The Extra Pharmacopoeia* (The Pharmaceutical Press, London), 26 ed., p. 377, 1972.

Mattison, J., Cannabis indica as an anodyne and hypnotic. *St. Louis Medical and Surgical Journal* 61:265–271 (1891).

Maugh, Thomas, Jr., Keys to body's pain control system found. *Los Angeles Times* Dec. 18:A-3 (1992).

Maurer, Henn, Dittrich, et al., Delta-9-THC shows antispastic and analgesic effects in a single case double-blind trial. *European Archive of Psychiatry and Clinical Neuroscience* 240:1–4 (1990).

Mauro, Tony, Legalize marijuana, prominent jurist says. *USA Today* Sept. 14 (1995).

Mayer-Gross, W., et al. *Clinical Psychiatry* (Cassell, London), 1969.

Mayor's Committee on Marihuana. *The Marihuana Problem in the City of New York: Sociological, Medical, Psychological and Pharmacological Studies* (Cattell Press, Lancaster, PA), 1944.

McCoy, Alfred, *The Politics of Heroin in Southeast Asia.*

Mechoulam & Feigenbaum, Progress towards cannabinoid drugs. *Medicinal Chemistry* 24:159–207 (1987).

Mechoulam R, Ed., *Cannabinoids as Therapeutic Agents* (CRC Press, Boca Raton, FL), 1986.

Mechoulam, R., Interview by David Pate. *Journal of the International Hemp Association* 1:21–23 (1994).

Mechoulam, R., Marihuana chemistry. *Science* June 5:1159–1166 (1970).

Meinck, Schonle, & Conrad, Effect of cannabinoids on spasticity and ataxia in MS. *Journal of Neurology* 236:120–122 (1989).

Melges, Tinklenberg, Hollister, & Gillespie, Marihuana and temporal disintegration. *Science* 168(3935):1118–1120 (1970).

Mendelson, Dr. Jack H., *New England Journal of Medicine* November (1974).

Merck Manual of Diagnosis and Therapy (Merck Pharmaceuticals, Rahway, NJ), 1992.

Mestel, R., Cannabis: The brain's other supplier. *New Scientist* July 31 (1993).

Meyer, R. E., Pillard, R. C., Mirin, S. M., Shapiro, L. S., & Fisher, S. Administration of marihuana to heavy and casual users. In *Minutes of American Psychiatric Association Meeting, Washington, DC, May 1971.*

Mikuriya, Tod H., Cannabis substitution, an adjunctive therapeutic tool in the treatment of alcoholism. *Medical Times* 98(4):187–191 (1970).

Mikuriya, Tod H., Marihuana in medicine, past, present and future. *California Medicine* 110:39–40 (1969).

Mikuriya, Tod H., Ed., *Marihuana: Medical Papers, 1839–1972* (Medi-Comp Press, Berkeley, CA), 1973.

Miller, C., & Wirtshafter, D., *Hemp Seed Cookbook* (Ohio Hempery, Inc.), 1992.

Miller, T. Q., *Psychological Bulletin* August (1996).

Miras, C. J., Some aspects of cannabis action. *Hashish: Its Chemistry and Pharmacology*, Wolstenholme & Knight, Eds. [Ciba Foundation 21] (J.&A. Churchill, London), 1965.

Molotosky, I., Animal antibiotics tied to illness in humans. *New York Times* Feb. 22 (1987).

Moore, Brent, *The Hemp Industry in Kentucky: A Study of the Past, the Present and the Possibilities* (Press of James E. Hughes, Lexington, KY), 1905.

Moreau de Tours, J. J., Lypemanie avec Stupeur: Tendence á la demence, traitement par l'extrait Guerison, resineux de cannabis indica. *Gazette des Hopitaux Civils et Militaires* 30:391 (1857).

Morgan, John P., Marijuana metabolism in the context of urine testing. *Journal of Psychoactive Drugs* 20(1):107–115 (1988).

Morton, Thomas, *New English Canaan*, p. 64, 1632.

Mott, Lawrie, & Snyder, Karen, *Pesticide Alert: A Guide to Pesticides in Fruits and Vegetables* (Natural Resources Defense Council, Sierra Club Books, San Francisco), 1987.

Musto, David F., *The American Disease: Origins of Narcotic Control* (Colonial Press, Clinton, MA), 1973.

National Academy of Science, *Biophysics and Biological Science Proceedings*, March 1983.

National Association of Attorneys General, *Therapeutic Use of Marijuana* (Committee on Criminal Law and Law Enforcement XI), by Vote of the Association Assembled, June 25, 1983.

National Commission on Marihuana and Drug Abuse, *Marihuana: A Signal of Misunderstanding* (New American Library, Inc., New York), 1972.

National Research Council, *Diet and Health: Implications for Reducing Chronic Disease Risk* (National Academy Press, Washington, DC), p. 57, 1989.

Navrátil, J., Effectiveness of *C. indica* in chronic otitis media. *Acta Univ.*

Palack. Olomuc. 6:87(1955) [in Czech.].

Nelson, Walsh, Deeter, et al., A phase II study of Δ-9-THC for appetite stimulation in cancer- associated anorexia. *Journal Palliative Care* 10(1):14–18 (1994).

Neu, Powers, King, & Gardner, Letter: Cannabis and chromosomes. *Lancet* 675 (1969).

Norman Goundry, translator, *Da Ma (Hemp. Marijuana—Cannabis sativa)* (Translations from the Ben Cao Gang Mu., Madeira Park, British Columbia), 1995.

Noyes Jr., R, Brunk, S. F., Avery, D. H., et al., The analgesic properties of Δ-9-THC and codeine. *Clinical Pharmacology Therapeutics* 18(1):84–89 (1975).

Ohlsson, et al., Plasma Δ-9-THC concentrations and clinical effects after oral and intravenous administration and smoking. *Clinical Pharmacology Therapeutics* 28:409 (1980).

Oliver, J., On the action of *Cannabis indica. British Medical Journal* 1:905–906 (1883).

Osburn, L., Hempseed, 2. *Hemp Line Journal* 1(2):12 (1992).

Osburn, L., Hempseed: The most nutritionally complete food in the world, 1. *Hemp Line Journal* 1(1):14 (1992).

O'Shaughnessy, W. B., Case of tetanus, cured by a preparation of hemp. *Translations of the Medical and Physical Society of Calcutta* 8:462–469 (1842).

O'Shaughnessy, W. B., On the Preparation of Indian Hemp, or Gunjah. *Translations of the Medical and Physical Society of Calcutta* 8(2):421–461 (1842).

Osler, W., & McCrae, T., *Principles and Practice of Medicine* (Appleton & Co., New York), 8th ed., p. 1089, 1916.

Ostrow, R., 48% of cancer specialists in study would prescribe pot. *Los Angeles Time* May 1:A-12 (1991).

Paine, Thomas, *Common Sense,* Pamphlet, 1776.

Pall of turmoil and concern over medical marijuana law good judgment of doctors is the only real protection for now. *Los Angeles Times* Nov. 10 (1996).

Panini, v. 2.29.

Parsons, Treatment of tetanus with cannabis indica. *Medical Times Gazette* 1 (1862).

Patnaik, Naveen, *The Garden of Life: An Introduction to the Healing Plants of India* (Doubleday Books, New York), pp. 8, 34, 1993.

Peat, Jones, et al., The disposition of Δ-9-THC in frequent and infrequent marijuana users. *Journal of Pharmacol. Exp. Therap.* (1987).

Petro, D., Marihuana as a therapeutic agent for muscle spasm or spasticity. *Psychosomatics* 21:81–85 (1980).

Petro, D., & Ellenberger, C., Treatment of human spasticity with Δ-9-THC. *Journal of Clinical Pharmacology* 21:413S–416S (1981).

Petwardhan, G. M., et al., Gas-chromatographic detection of resins in cannabis seeds. *Indian Journal of Pharmaceutical Sciences* 40(5):166–167 (1978).

Pimentel, D., Energy and land constraints in food protein production. *Science* Nov. 21 (1975).

Pimentel, David & Marcia, *Food, Energy and Society,* 59 (1979).

Piomelli, Daniele, et al., *Nature* Aug. 22 (1996).

Plinius Secundus, Caius, *De Historia Natura,* 20.97.

Purvis, J. P., *Through Uganda to Mt. Elgon* (Fisher Unwin, London), pp. 336–337, 1909.

Radosevic, A., Kupinic, M., & Grlic, L., Antibiotic activity of various types of cannabis resin. *Nature* 195:1007–1009.

Randall, R. C., *Cancer Treatment and Marijuana Therapy* (Galen Press, Washington, DC), 1990.

Randall, R. C., Ed., *Marijuana, Medicine and the Law* (Galen Press, Washington, DC), Vol. I, 1988; Vol. II, 1991.

Rathbun, Mary, & Peron, Dennis, *Brownie Mary's Marijuana Cookbook and Dennis Peron's Recipe for Social Change* (Trail of Smoke Publishing, San Francisco), 1993.

Regelson, W., Butler, J. R, Schultz, J., et al., Δ-9-THC as an effective antidepressant and appetite stimulating agent in advanced cancer patients. In *Proceedings of the International Conference Pharmacology Cannabis*, M. C. Braude and S. Szara, Eds. (Raven Press, Savannah, GA),1975.

Rennie, S. J., On the therapeutic value of tincture cannabis indica in the treatment of dysentery: More particularly in its subacute and chronic forms. *Indian Medical Gazette* 21:353–355 (1886).

Report of the President's Advisory Commission on Narcotics and Drug Abuse, 1963.

Resenberg, B., Curb on U.S. waste urged to help the world's hungry. *New York Times* Oct. 25 (1974).

Reuters, Hole in ozone layer is bigger than ever, UN official says. *San Francisco Chronicle* Nov. 28:B-4 (1996).

Reynolds, J. R., Therapeutic uses and toxic effects of *Cannabis indica. Lancet* 1:637–638 (1900).

Rg Veda., ix. 61.13.

Richardson, Day, & Taylor, Effect of prenatal alcohol, marijuana and tobacco exposure on neonatal behavior. *Infant Behavior and Development* 12(2):199–209 (1989).

Ritchie, J. M., The aliphatic alcohols. In *The Pharmacological Basis of Therapeutics,* Goodman & Gilman, Eds. (Macmillan, New York), 3rd. ed., Chap. 11, pp. 143–153, 1965.

Robbe, H., & O'Hanlon, J., *HS 808 078: Marijuana and Actual Driving Performance* (U.S. Department of Transportation, National Technical Information Service, Springfield VA), p. 1, 1993.

Robbins, J., *Environmental Impact Resulting from Unconfined Animal Production* (EPA Environmental Research Information Center, Cincinnati,

OH), Environmental Protection Technology Series, p. 9, February 1978.

Robbins, John, *Diet for a New America* (Stillpoint Publishing, Walpole, NH), pp. 330, 353, 1987.

Robinson, Rowan, *The Great Book of Hemp* (Inner Traditions, Rochester, VT), 1996.

Rodin, E., Domino, E. F., & Porzak, J. P., The marihuana-induced 'social high'—Neurological and electroencephalographic concomitants. *Journal of the American Medical Association* 213:1300–1302 (1970).

Rolls, E. J., & Stafford-Clark, D., Depersonalization treated by *Cannabis indica* and psychotherapy. *Guy's Hospital Reports* 103:330–336 (1954).

Rosen, Dr. Max, *Journal of Urology* May (1991).

Rosenburg, C. M., The use of marijuana in the treatment of alcoholism. In *The Therapeutic Potential of Marijuana*, Cohen & Stillman, Eds. (Plenum Medical Book Pub., New York), pp. 173–85, 1976.

Rosenthal, Ed, Logan, William, & Steinborn, Jeffery, *Marijuana: The Law and You—A Guide to Minimizing Legal Consequences* (Quick American Archives), 1995.

Rubin, Dr. Vera, & Comitas, Lambros, *Ganja in Jamaica: A Medical Anthropological Study of Chronic Marijuana Use* (Mouton & Co./Anchor Books, New York), 1975.

Sackett & Hobbs, *Hemp: A War Crop* (Mason & Hanger Co., New York), 1942.

Sagan, Carl, *The Dragons of Eden* (H&J Publishing, London), 1977.

Salladay, Robert, Lungren lays down medical pot law. *Oakland Tribune* Dec. 4:A-7 (1996).

Sallan, Cronin, Zelen, & Zinberg, Antiemetics in patients receiving chemotherapy for cancer. *New England Journal of Medicine* 302:135–138 (1980).

Sallan, S. E., Zinberg, N. E., & Frei, III, E., Antiemetic effect of Δ-9-THC in patients receiving cancer chemotherapy. *New England Journal of Medicine* 293(16):795–797 (1975).

San Francisco Chronicle March 24:11 (1996).

San Francisco Chronicle Nov. 10:7 (1996).

San Francisco Chronicle Sept. 28 (1996).

Sandyk & Awerbuch, Letter: Marijuana and Tourette's Syndrome. *Journal of Clinical Psycho. Pharmacology* 8(6):444–445 (1988).

Sandyk, Consroe, Stern, & Snider, Effects of CBD in Huntington's disease. *Neurology* 36(Suppl. 1):342 (1986).

Sasman, Marty, Cannabis indica in pharmaceuticals. *Journal of the New Jersey Medical Society* 35:51–52 (1938).

Scarlett, R. G. [W.G. Scarlett Corp. of Baltimore, MD], *Transcript of the Hearing on HR 6385*, Committee on Ways and Means, House of Representatives, 75c 1s. April 27–30, May 4, 1937.

Scher, Richardson, et al., Effects of prenatal alcohol and marijuana exposure. *Pediatric Research* 24(1)101–105 (1988).

Schofield, M., *The Strange Case of Pot* (Penguin Books, Middlesex, England), p. 17, 1971.

Scientists advocate marijuana for the ill. *Reuter* Nov. 15 (1994).

Segal, THC as an analgesic for pain relief. *IHA Journal* (1986).

Should the world go to pot? *New Times* [San Luis Obispo, CA] Feb. 7:14–15 (1991).

Silberman, Buckley, & Henderson, Circuit Judges. *In the Matter of Marijuana Rescheduling Petition*, Ninth circuit court of appeals, April 1991.

Silver, Beth, Deformed frogs alarm students, scientists. *San Francisco Examiner* Oct. 10:A-1 (1996).

Silverstein, M.J., & Lessin, P. J., Normal skin test responses in chronic marihuana users. *Science* 186:740–741 (1974).

Sim, V., Proceedings of a Workshop on Psychotomimetic Drugs. In *Psychotomimetic Drugs*, D. Efron, Ed. (Raven Press, New York), 1970.

Sloman, Larry, *The History of Marijuana in America: Reefer Madness* (Bobbs–Merrill Company, Indianapolis, IN), pp. 152–158, 1979.

Small, Beckstead, & Chan, The evolution of cannabinoid phenotypes in cannabis. *Economic Botany* 29:219–232 (1975).

Smoked marijuana called effective remedy. *Boston Globe* June 28:12 (1991).

Smoking to live. *60 Minutes* (CBS News), 24:11. Dec. 1 (1991).

Snyder, Solomon H., *Uses of Marijuana* (Oxford University Press, Toronto), 1971.

Snyder, Solomon H., What have we forgotten about pot? *New York Times Magazine* Dec. 13:26 (1970).

Soderstrom, Triffilis, Shankar, Clark, & Cowley, Marijuana and alcohol use among 1023 trauma patients. *Archives of Survey* 123:733–737 (1988).

Spyker, Dan. CDER Research Proposal RFP: Multicenter single-patient randomized clinical trials of Δ-9-THC, Submitted for publication, 1991.

St. Angelo, J., et al., Isolation of edestin from aleurone grains of *Cannabis sativa*. *Archives of Biochemistry and Biophysics* 124:199–205 (1968).

Starks, Michael, *Marijuana Chemistry: Genetics, Processing and Potency* (Ronin Publishing, Berkeley, CA), 2nd ed., 1990.

Stockings, G. T., A new euphoriant for depressive mental states. *British Medical Journal*, 918–922 (1947).

Stockwell, M., et al., Chromatography of edestin at 50 degrees, *Biochimica et Biophysica Acta* 82:221–230 (1964).

Strawn, N., Alcohol fuels: Alternatives for today and the future. *Biologue* September:13–16 (1990).

Suckling, C. W., On the therapeutic value of Indian hemp. *British Medical Journal* 11:12. July 4 (1891).

Summary Report, 1987 National Resources Inventory. *Statistical Bulletin 790* December (1989) [USDA Soil Conservation Service].

Susruta samhita, Kalpa 15:5, Sutra 15:41.7th C. bc.

Tashkin, D. P., Shapiro, B. J., & Frank. I. A., Acute pulmonary physiologic effects of smoked marihuana and oral Δ-9-THC in healthy young men. *New England Journal of Medicine* 289:336–341 (1973).

Tashkin, et al., Marijuana Pulmonary Research (University of California, Los Angeles), 1969–1983.

Tashkin, Shapiro, Lee, & Harper, Effects of smoked marihuana in experimentally induced asthma. *American Review of Respiratory Disease* 112:377–386 (1975).

Tashkin, Wu, Djahed, & Rose, Marijuana and tobacco: Comparative hazards. *Brown University Digest of Addiction Theory and Application* 7(3):29 (1988).

Tennes, Avitable, et al., Marijuana: Prenatal and postnatal exposure in the human. *NIDA Monograph Series* 113:48–60 (1985).

Teramura, Alan, *Discover* September (1989).

Thompson, L. J., & Proctor, R. C., The use of pyrahexyl in the treatment of alcoholic and drug withdrawal conditions. *North Carolina Medical Journal* 14:520–523 (1953).

Toxic ten, *Mother Jones* January:40(1993).

Two drugs approved for AIDS, *Washington Post* Dec. 24:A-5(1992).

United Nations, *Charter of the United Nations* (New York), Preamble, Article 2, 1946.

United Nations, *Single Convention Treaty on Narcotic Drugs* (United Nations, New York), Preamble, Article 28, 1961, 1968.

United Nations, *Universal Declaration on Human Rights* (United Nations, New York), Article 25.1, 1948.

U.S. Department of Agriculture, *The Official Record* Dec. 25:3 (1930).

U.S. v. Randall, 104 Washington, DC Superior Court, Daily Law report 2249, 1976.

U.S. v. Timothy Leary, U.S. Supreme Court.

U.S. Senate, *Transcript of the hearing before a subcommittee of the Committee on Finance* (Library of Congress), 75c 2s, HR 6906, July 12, 1937.

van der Werf, Hayo, *Crop Physiology of Fibre Hemp* (Proefschrift Wageningen, Wageningen University, The Netherlands), 1994.

Van Klingeren and Ten Ham, THC's antibacterial properties. IHA Journal (1976).

Vichery, Smith, & Nolan, Connecticut agricultural experiment station: A substitute for edestin. *Science* 92:317–318 (1940).

Vinciguerra, V., Moore, T., & Brennan, E., Inhalation marijuana as an antiemetic for cancer chemotherapy. *New York State Journal of Medicine* October:525–527 (1988).

Wallach, Leah, The chemistry of reefer madness. *Omni* August:18 (1989).

Walton, R., *Marijuana: America's New Drug Problem* (Lippincott, Philadelphia, PA), 1938.

Warning: Unsafe for human life, *Longevity* August 22 (1991).

Washington Post Service, EPA study reinforces link between dioxin and cancer. *Buffalo News* [New York] Sept. 12 (1994).

Washington Post Service, Night goggles illuminate military's drug role. *Oakland Tribune* Nov. 30:A-6 (1996).

Waskow, Olsson, Salzman, & Katz, Psychological effects of THC. *Review of General Psychiatry* 22(2):97–107 (1970).

Watt, J. M., & Breyer-Brandwijk, M. G., *The Medicinal and Poisonous Plants of Southern Africa* (E&S Livingstone, Edinburgh, Scotland), 1932.

Weil, A. T., Zinberg, N. E., & Nelsen, J. M., Clinical and psychological effects of marihuana in man. *Science* 162:1234–1242 (1968).

Weil, Andrew, & Rosen, Winifred, *From Chocolate to Morphine* (Houghton Mifflin, Boston, MA), 1993.

Weil, Andrew, Therapeutic Hemp Oil. *Natural Health* March/April:10–12 (1993).

Weiner, Michael & Janet, *Herbs That Heal* (Quantum Books, Mill Valley, CA), pp. 225–226, 1994.

Weiss, B. L., Coptic Study, Ethiopian Zion Coptic Church, Florida, 1980.

West, M. E. [University of West Indies, Kingston, Jamaica], Letter, *Nature* July (1991).

Wikler, A., & Lloyd, B. J., Effect of smoking marihuana cigarettes on cortical electrical activity. *Federation Proceedings* 4 :141–142 (1945).

Wilson, C., More thoughts on why pot is a drag. *San Francisco Examiner* Nov. 1:C-21 (1996).

Wood, G. B., & Bache, F., *Dispensatory of the United States* (Lippincott, Brambo & Co., Philadelphia, PA), p. 339, 1854.

Would you still rather fight than switch? *Whole Life Times* April–May (1985).

Yearbook of the U.S. Department of Agriculture 1930 (Washington, DC), 1931.

Yoga Sutra, IV:I.

Young, Francis L. [DEA Administrative Law Judge], *In the Matter of Marijuana Rescheduling Petition,* Docket No 86-22, Sept. 6, 1988.

Zand, Janet, Walton, Rachel, & Roundtree, Bob, *Smart Medicine for a Healthier Child* (Avery Publishing Group, Garden City Park, NY), pp. 3–75, 432–434, 1994.

Zias, J., et al., Early medical use of cannabis. *Nature* May 20:215 (1993).

Zuardi, A. W., Shirakawa, I., Finkelfarb, E., & Karniol, I.G., Action of cannabidiol on the anxiety and other effects produced by Δ9–THC in normal subjects. *Psychopharacology* 76:245–250 (1982).

Zuardi, A. W., Rodrigues, J. A., Cunha, J. M., Effects of CBD in animal models predictive of anti-psychotic activity. *Psychopharmacology* 104:260–264 (1991).

Zuckerman, Frank, et al., Effects of maternal marijuana and cocaine use on fetal growth. *New England Journal of Medicine* 320(12):7652–768 (1989).

Index